THE CLIMBING BIBLE

MANAGING INJURIES

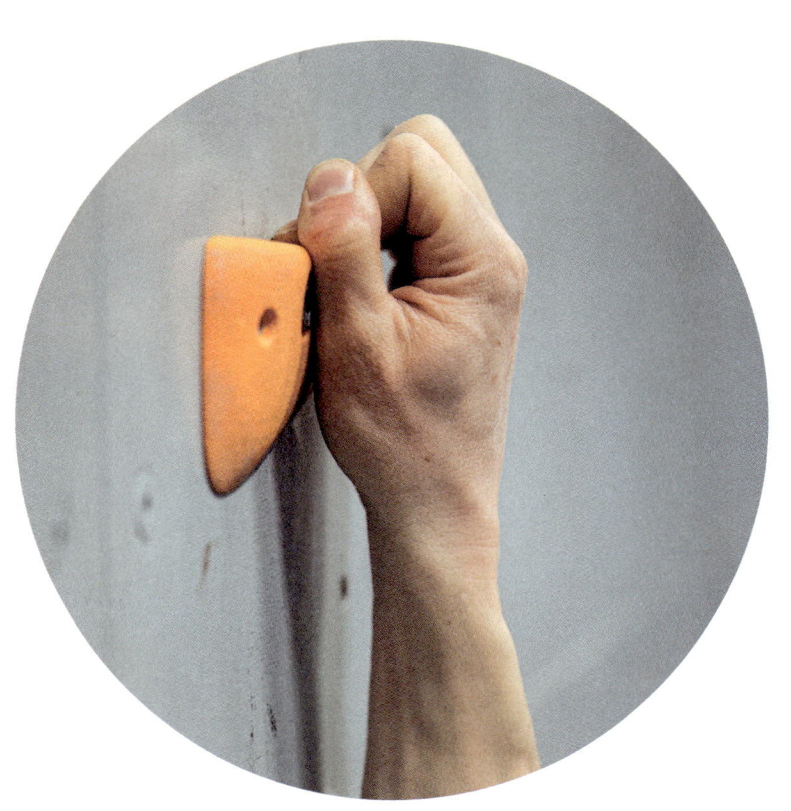

THE CLIMBING BIBLE

MANAGING INJURIES

INJURY PREVENTION AND REHABILITATION
FOR CLIMBING AND BOULDERING

STIAN CHRISTOPHERSEN

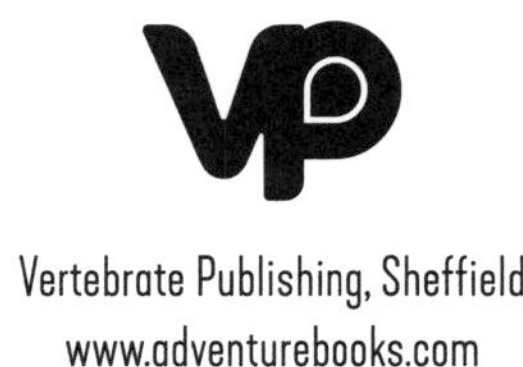

Vertebrate Publishing, Sheffield
www.adventurebooks.com

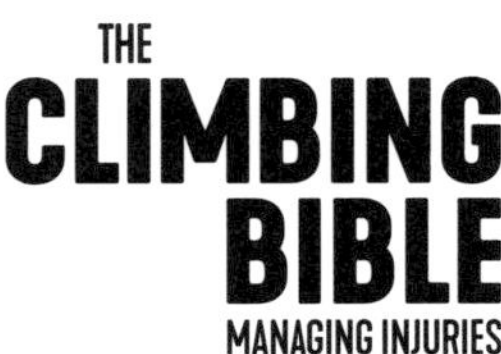

STIAN CHRISTOPHERSEN

First published simultaneously in English and Norwegian in 2024 by Vertebrate Publishing and Klatreboka AS.

The author has received support from the Norwegian Non-Fiction Writers and Translators Association.

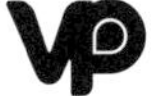
Vertebrate Publishing
Omega Court, 352 Cemetery Road, Sheffield S11 8FT, United Kingdom.
www.adventurebooks.com

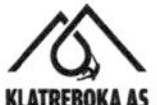

Cover photography by Bård Lie Henriksen; cover illustrations by Dr Joanna Butler.
Photography by Bård Lie Henriksen unless otherwise credited.
Medical illustrations by Dr Joanna Butler, Medical Artist Ltd. *www.medical-artist.com*
Edited by John Coefield. Design by Jon Tore Modell.

A CIP catalogue record for this book is available from the British Library.

ISBN: 978-1-83981-200-2 (Paperback)
ISBN: 978-1-83981-201-9 (Ebook)

10 9 8 7 6 5 4 3 2 1

Vertebrate Publishing is committed to printing on paper from sustainable sources.

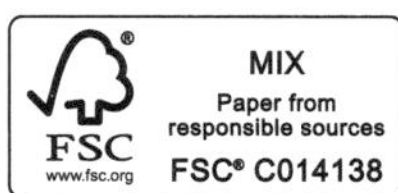

Printed and bound in Slovenia by Latitude Press.

CONTENTS

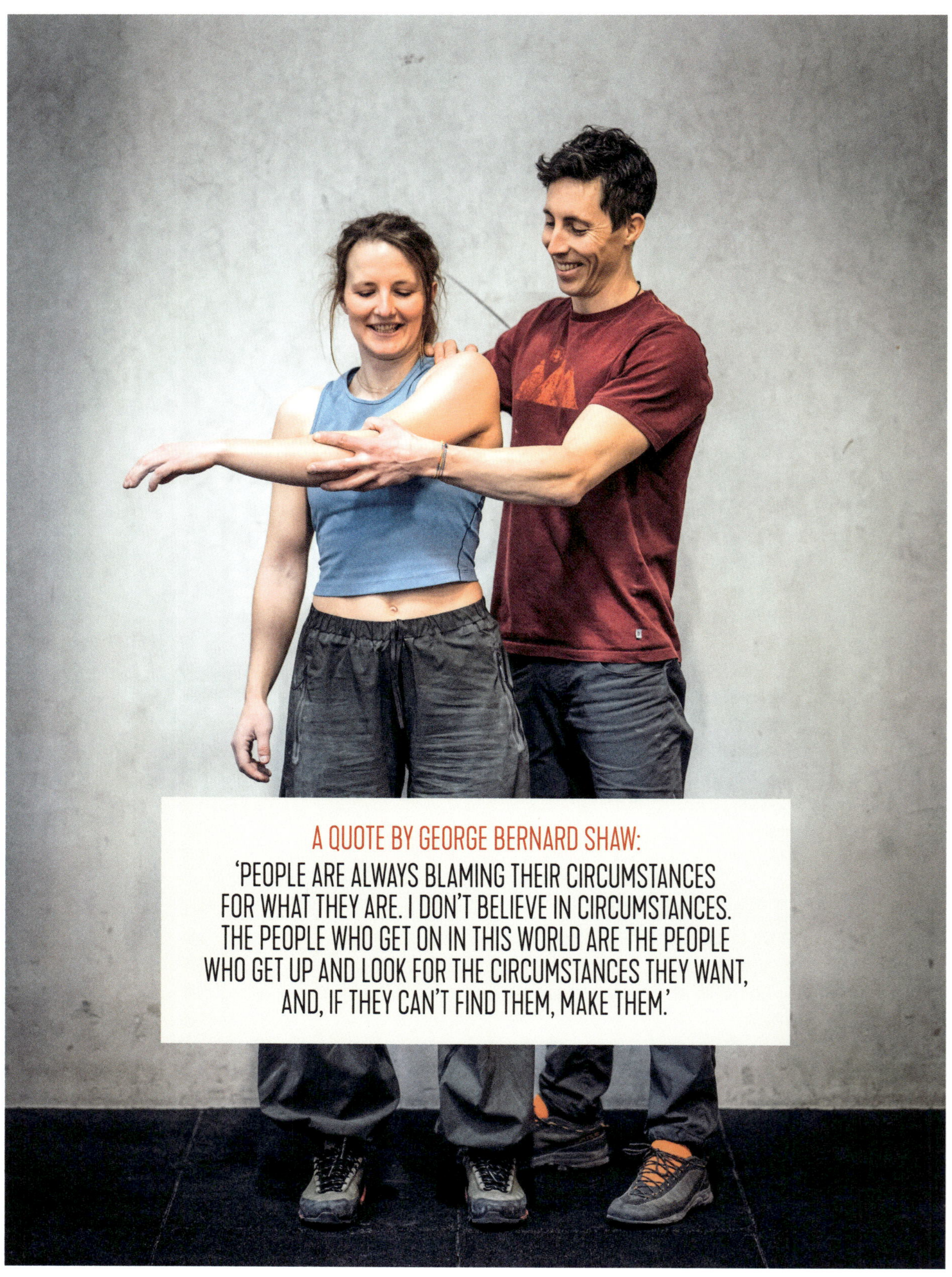

A QUOTE BY GEORGE BERNARD SHAW:

‘PEOPLE ARE ALWAYS BLAMING THEIR CIRCUMSTANCES FOR WHAT THEY ARE. I DON’T BELIEVE IN CIRCUMSTANCES. THE PEOPLE WHO GET ON IN THIS WORLD ARE THE PEOPLE WHO GET UP AND LOOK FOR THE CIRCUMSTANCES THEY WANT, AND, IF THEY CAN’T FIND THEM, MAKE THEM.’

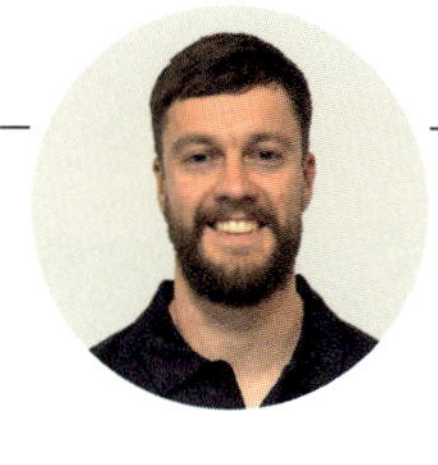

FOREWORD

JAMES WALKER

PHYSIOTHERAPIST AND CLIMBER, SHEFFIELD CLIMBING CLINIC

Many climbing injuries, such as finger pulley injuries, are unique to climbing in the sense that they don't occur in any other sports. Even with the injuries that do occur in both climbing and other sports – for example, a shoulder dislocation – there is a unique demand placed on the injured area for the climber to successfully return to climbing. No other sport requires a cut loose to a sloper, or a foot match while in an overhead gaston position! It is therefore vital that a clinician involved in the rehabilitation of climbing injuries understands not only the injury but the sport too.

Moreover, climbing is a lifestyle sport. For many climbers, it is more than just a hobby. It is therefore essential that a clinician understands the significant effect that being injured can have on a climber and the importance to them of moving forwards and returning to climbing as efficiently as possible.

I first met Stian a few years ago after he contacted me with the idea of starting a podcast all about climbing injuries. A few months later he was travelling to the UK for work and we met in person on a glorious, crisp, cold, sunny day at a boulder in the Burbage Valley in the Peak District near where I live. Later that day over dinner, the idea for the *Climbing Injury Podcast* was born.

We've spoken regularly over the last few years, either when recording the podcast or just chatting about climbing. One thing that shines through is Stian's passion for climbing. His knowledge of climbing injuries and the mechanics of climbing itself is excellent, and it is clear how much he cares about getting his patients back on the wall. As climbing is more than just a hobby for many climbers, you can tell that being a climbing physiotherapist is more than just a job for Stian.

Stian has also climbed at the highest level and picked up – and successfully recovered from – multiple injuries. This personal understanding of what it takes to get to a high level of climbing as well as to come back from injury really helps in the process of rehabilitating other climbers.

As a climbing physiotherapist myself I have seen the sport change massively over the years. Climbing's popularity – especially bouldering – around the world, has skyrocketed, and with climbing now in its second Olympics and confirmed for its third, this popularity will most likely continue to increase. And an increase in participation of climbing will likely result in an increased number of climbing injuries.

Compared to other sports, research into the management of climbing injuries is tiny. Some of the research that has been done is excellent, however there is often a lack of specificity when it comes to the rehabilitation of an injury.

What Stian has done with this book is provide a fantastic resource for both climbers and clinicians working with climbers to use as guidance for rehabilitation of the most common climbing injuries. I can envision this book sitting on the shelf of climbers' homes and being used to give them an understanding of what the tweak they have picked up could be.

Well done to Stian for writing this book and helping to push forward the knowledge base around climbing injuries.

Happy climbing – I just hope that the number of chapters in this book you require isn't too high!

INTRODUCTION: THE PURPOSE OF THIS BOOK

When I was 16 years old, I had only been climbing for two years and yet I already defined myself as a climber – much of my identity revolved around being good at climbing, even though I wasn't climbing anywhere near what was then the international competition level. My social circle mostly consisted of climbers: it was where my best friends and role models were, and where I felt most comfortable and accepted. The desire to become much better than I was at that time was strong; I trained obsessively and with purpose, climbing almost every day.

I don't remember exactly when it started, but one day I began experiencing pain in the middle (PIP) joints of both middle fingers. The joints would swell after training, be stiff in the morning and be painful to touch. Experiencing pain while taking part in sport is not uncommon, so I assumed this would eventually go away. But it didn't. After a few months, I went to see a doctor who gave me an anti-inflammatory ointment and advised me to take it easy. Without receiving a specific answer about what this finger problem could be, taking it easy was out of the question for me; the junior world championships were coming up in a few months' time and making a tough decision not to climb would require much clearer advice and information than what I had been given.

A month later, I went to see another doctor and got similar results there too: no clear answers, but encouragement to rest until the issue resolved itself. So, despite having painful fingers, I continued training while applying ointment to the joints and hoping that they would get better over time.

A few months later, doctor number three decided to X-ray my fingers. When the results came back, he informed me that I had stress fractures – essentially broken bones – in the growth plates of both middle fingers. He clearly instructed me not to climb for the next six weeks, but also advised me to train everything else that didn't strain my fingers. Most importantly, he assured me that if I did this correctly, the injury would fully heal and not bother me again in the future. I skipped the junior world championships and took it relatively easy for those six weeks, doing alternative training during that summer; I never had any problems with that injury again.

This little story from 25 years ago has taught me a lot – both about athletes and healthcare professionals. About what athletes are willing to go through regardless of their level to engage in an activity they love. About the significance of the type of person they encounter among healthcare professionals when seeking help for their injuries and ailments. And about what knowledge and information is needed and available, and how it is communicated between healthcare professionals and their patients.

Looking back, it's obvious that we now have much more knowledge about climbing-related injuries than we did 25 years ago. We also have much more knowledge about sports injuries in general. So, even though the occurrence of climbing-related injuries is increasing with the growing numbers of new climbers, we – healthcare professionals, coaches and parents – have a better understanding of how to address these injuries, both in reducing the risk of injury in the first place, and managing them when they occur.

Klatre-talent fester NM-grepet

«Det stilles stadig større krav til styrke. Hvert «flytt» er ganske krevende»
Stian Christophersen

Stadig oppover. Stian Christophersen jager mot toppen. 18-åringen hører til klatre-eliten her i landet.

METTE BUGGE
OLAV URDAHL (foto)

NM-favoritt. Unggutten fra Brønnøya i Asker er villig til å satse hardt for å få et skikkelig grep om denne sporten. NM-gull under mesterskapet i Kongsberg i juniorklassen i kveld er første mål, men han stiller også i seniorklassen i morgen. Der regner han med at kameraten Martin Mobråten (19), også han fra Asker, blir den sterkeste.

– Jeg klatrer på sjette året, forteller Stian.

Han legger til at han ble helt hektet på denne sporten fra første stund. Pappa var turklatrer. Stian er sportsklatrer som mener at veggene innendørs er mest utfordrende.

– Det gjelder å ha pump, sier Stian. *«Pump» er utholdenhet på klatrespråket. Stian har det, og dessuten styrke og forståelse av hvordan en rute bør legges opp.*

– Det stilles stadig større krav til styrke. Hvert «flytt» er ganske krevende, forklarer han.

Under NM får deltagerne fem minutter til å se gjennom ruta før de skal i aksjon. Da gjelder det fort å finne ut hvordan det lønner seg å flytte armer og ben.

– Mange tror at det gjelder å komme fortest opp til toppen, men det gjelder å komme lengst.

I idrettstroppen

– Idretten er veldig allsidig, kommer det fra tenåringen som tidligere spilte fotball i Nesbru og deretter Holmen. Han ble lei av å møte opp til faste tider. Han ville kjøre sitt eget løp, men det betyr ikke at han sluntrer unna treningen. Stian Christophersen er med i idrettstroppen på Kolsås, og når han er ferdig med militæret i desember, bærer det ut i den store verden.

– Jeg og Martin kommer til å dra utenlands for å klatre mye, både i Spania og Frankrike.

Klatresenteret Tyrili i Oslo er hjemmebane for askerbøringen. Der får han god støtte av Miguel de Freitas, tidligere norsk landslagstrener, opprinnelig fra Portugal.

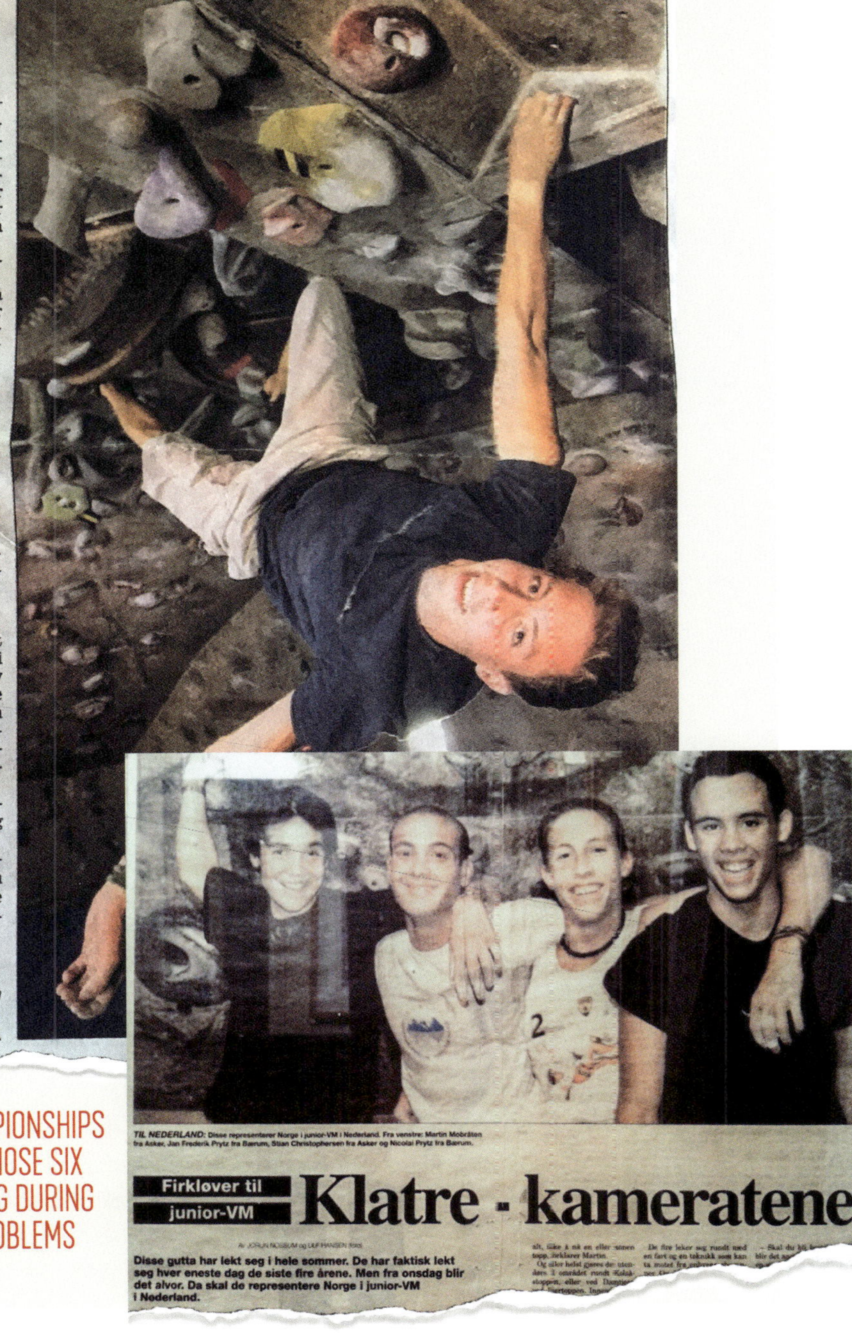

Grepa kar. *Stian Christophersen henger høyt, men er blid. Forberedelsene til NM har foregått på Tyrili.*

TIL NEDERLAND: Disse representerer Norge i junior-VM i Nederland. Fra venstre: Martin Mobråten fra Asker, Jan Frederik Prytz fra Bærum, Stian Christophersen fra Asker og Nicolai Prytz fra Bærum.

Firkløver til junior-VM

Klatre - kameratene

Disse gutta har lekt seg i hele sommer. De har faktisk lekt seg hver eneste dag de siste fire årene. Men fra onsdag blir det alvor. Da skal de representere Norge i junior-VM i Nederland.

'I SKIPPED THE JUNIOR WORLD CHAMPIONSHIPS AND TOOK IT RELATIVELY EASY FOR THOSE SIX WEEKS, DOING ALTERNATIVE TRAINING DURING THAT SUMMER; I NEVER HAD ANY PROBLEMS WITH THAT INJURY AGAIN.'

Unfortunately, when one wants to improve in a sport, injuries are a part of the game. A preventive measure can at best reduce the risk of an injury occurring, but even if we do everything right, there is still an element of chance involved. However, having more accessible knowledge can allow us to train more effectively with a generally lower level of risk; we can also recover more quickly if and when we do pick up an injury.

The aim of this book is to make a central contribution to the knowledge base that healthcare professionals can refer to when treating climbers, and also be understandable to climbers who do not have a medical background. Therefore, it will attempt to ride two horses simultaneously – by being scientifically strong yet presented simply – so that it is a valuable tool for both healthcare professionals and climbers.

I've always been fascinated by how our bodies work, but, perhaps more importantly, I've always been fascinated by working with people. After nearly 30 years as a climber – competing nationally and internationally; climbing outdoors all over the world; clinically treating patients for 15 years; training and medically managing athletes of all ages and levels, including the international elite; and writing two books on climbing training – I still feel the joy of developing myself as a professional in my field *and* as a climber.

This is why I felt it was time to write about the part of my work that deals with climbing injuries. Injuries that climbers get. Climbers who are people. People who consist not only of structural, biological and physiological aspects, but also thoughts, emotions, worries, joys and a sense of social belonging.

Therefore, this book is not solely a medical reference guide covering all of the climbing-related injuries described in scientific literature. Instead, it describes the most common climbing injuries and ailments that I encounter frequently in my clinical practice – and how they can be diagnosed and treated, and hopefully prevented. I examine these injuries from various perspectives – anatomical, physiological, psychological – encompassing topics such as the specific structures involved in injuries, pain physiology, overall load, exposure and movement optimism. The goal is for this book to collectively address all of the different factors that affect an individual who is experiencing pain or injury.

It's important to note that in all research and knowledge, there is a recurring issue that fixed protocols do not have the same effect on every individual who undergoes them. The same training protocol might be positive for some, negative for others, and some people might not experience any change at all. There can be many reasons for this, but the most important is that every person is different and unique in their own situation. A rehabilitation protocol or treatment method that works for me may not work for you. Therefore, I will be very cautious about presenting such protocols and methods as *universal* solutions; yet these protocols and methods are usually based on fundamental principles. So, if we understand the principles well enough, we can adapt the methods to fit an individual. That's why this book is based on such principles – so that the methods I've presented can become suggestions that you can customise to make them work specifically for you. I know it would be easier with a definitive answer and, if I had one, I would gladly give it to you, but we need to be humble regarding what we can actually say and claim.

This is a self-help book – a self-help book based on the best available knowledge and my personal and others' experiences from many years of climbing. It is a book for anyone involved in climbing, with or without a medical background, with the goal of reducing injury risk and helping climbers handle their injuries as effectively as possible when incidents do occur.

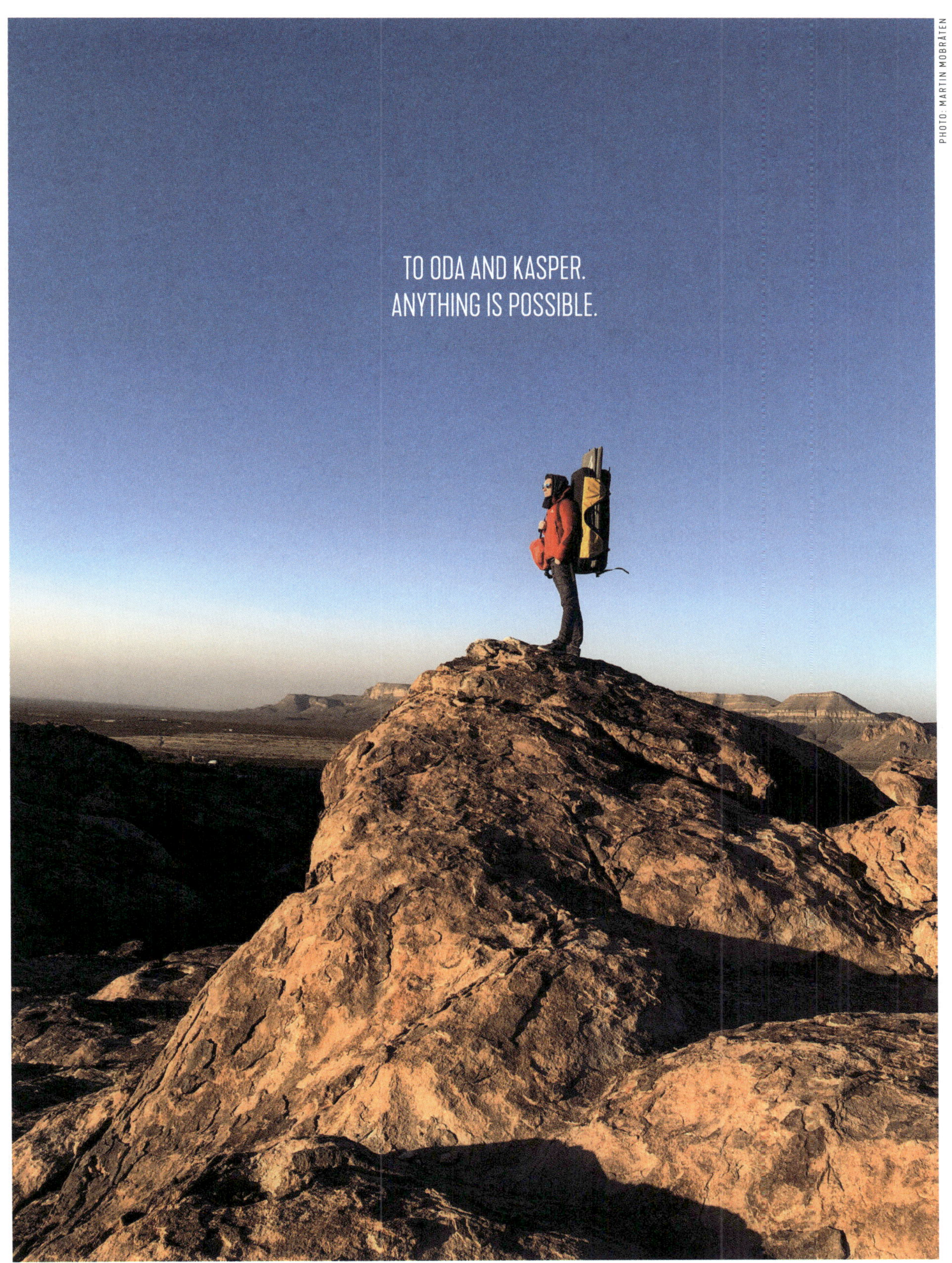

PHOTO: MARTIN MOBRÅTEN

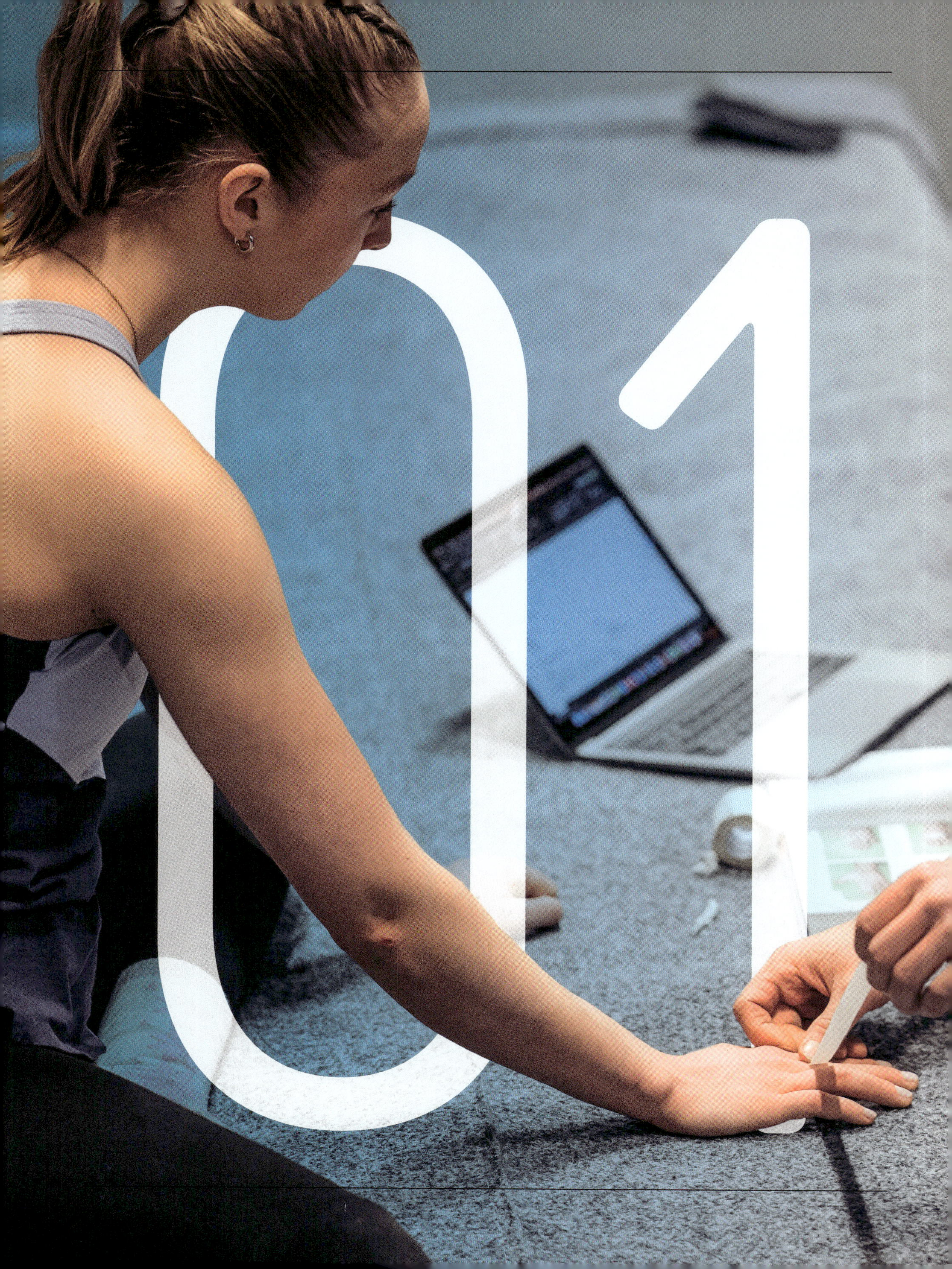
01

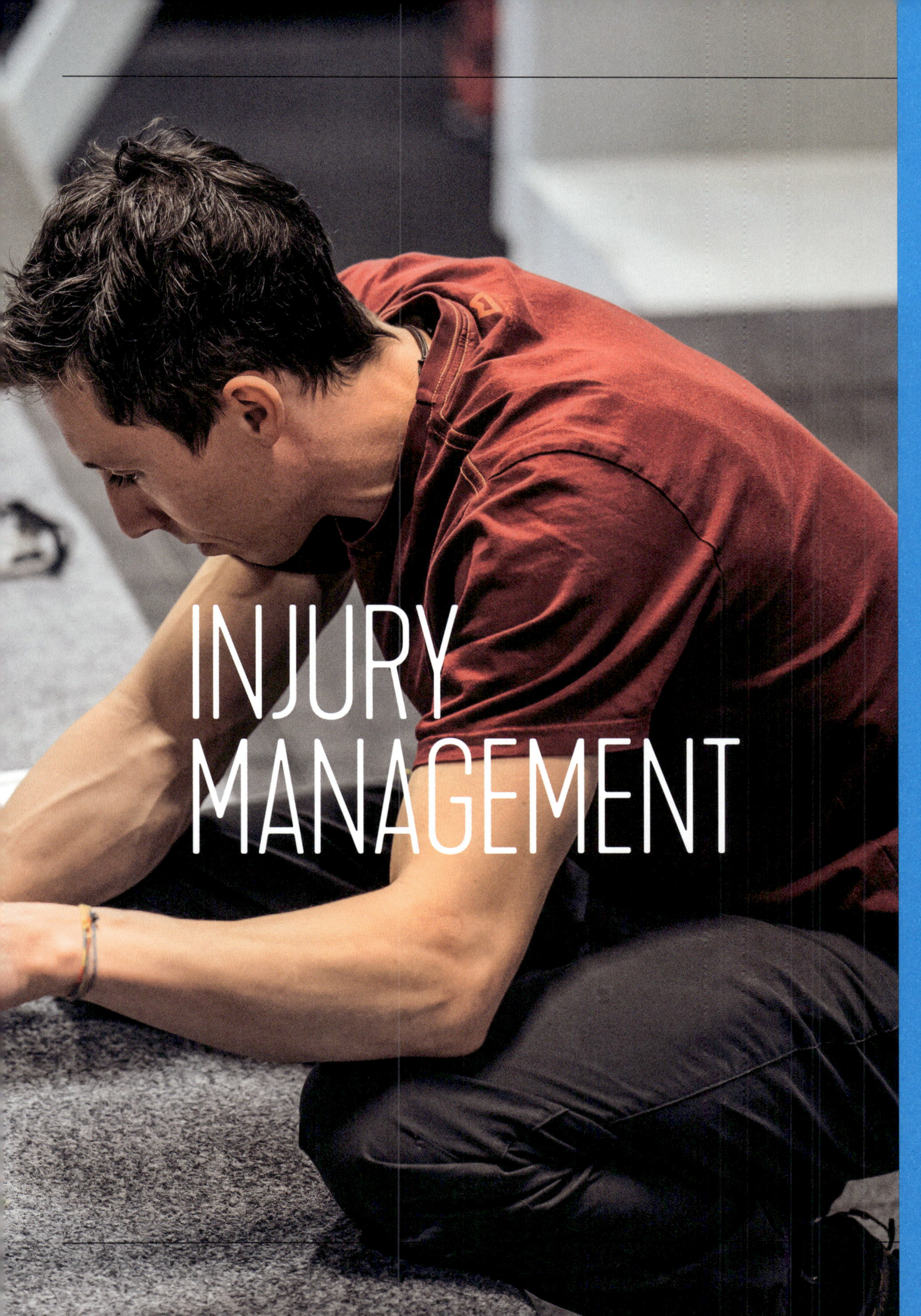

INJURY MANAGEMENT

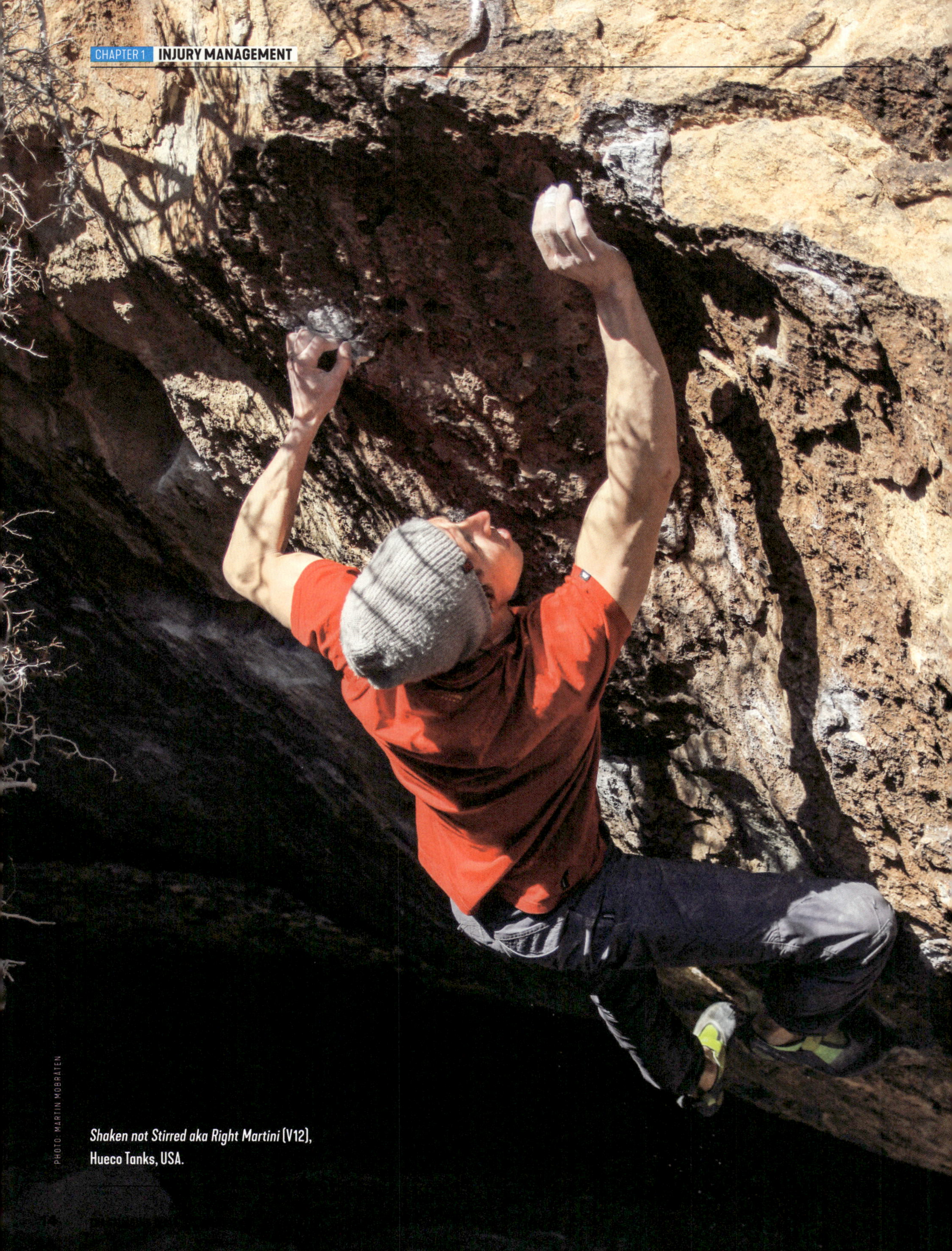

PHOTO: MARTIN MOBRATEN

Shaken not Stirred aka Right Martini (V12), Hueco Tanks, USA.

HANDLING OF ACUTE SOFT TISSUE INJURIES AND OVERUSE INJURIES

We differentiate between acute injuries and overuse injuries because these different types of injuries require different approaches to treatment. However, there are some common factors for treatment and prevention, and in this chapter we will look at the management of acute injuries and overuse injuries from various perspectives.

We will examine the principles for managing acute injuries, and look at how physiological, psychological and social factors affect injuries; factors such as load management, strength training, recovery, sleep and nutrition. This chapter lays the foundation for chapter 2 which looks at specific climbing-related injuries (page 38).

ACUTE SOFT TISSUE INJURIES

FEBRUARY 2019. *It is my last day in Hueco Tanks. I have never been to a better bouldering area. We have climbed a lot, and my body has taken a beating over the last ten days. Nevertheless, I feel good and ready to crush today's wishlist on East Mountain. After a quick – too quick – warm-up I go for a flash attempt on Mo Mojo (V11/8a), but fail miserably. I work through the sequence; the crux is pinching hard with my right hand while placing a high left heel hook by my left hand before deadpointing up to a left hand sidepull. The heel hook is high and close to my body, and I can feel that I really need to pull on it to get my body around the roof that the problem climbs along. However, it feels like something I've done hundreds of times before, so my surprise is great when on my next attempt I hear three distinct pops from my left hip and find myself sitting on the pad below.*

'What happened?' my friends ask.

I don't have an answer at the moment because, honestly, I don't feel much pain. Endorphins have that effect on us.

'Did you hear that?' I reply, as I check if my left hip is still where it should be.

It's the start of the last day, so it would take a lot for me to stop climbing today. And there isn't really any pain. I ignore the sneaking suspicion of a hamstring injury and move on to the next boulder. After a long day of climbing, a sandstorm forces us back to the car, and only then do I notice that I am limping. The next day, my left thigh is stiff all the way up to my buttock. The flight home from El Paso to Oslo is truly one for the books. Back home, what I initially suspected is confirmed. An injury in the hamstring muscles and tendon attachment at the sitting bone.

When tissues in our bodies are suddenly exposed to forces they cannot withstand, they become damaged to varying degrees. This tissue damage undergoes a healing process through three phases – *inflammation* phase, *repair* phase and *remodelling* phase – where the outcome of each phase affects both the next phase and the final outcome. This means that we actually want inflammation – an inflammatory response – even though, over the years, many hypotheses and models have been proposed which support the suppression of this response.

In this book we will focus on soft tissue injuries – injuries related to muscles, tendons and ligaments. Bone tissue injuries, such as acute fractures or stress fractures, are approached differently, primarily through stabilisation and immobilisation to ensure proper healing and stability.

In 1978, Dr Gabe Mirkin introduced RICE – Rest Ice Compression Elevation – as an acronym for managing acute injuries, with its goal being to reduce swelling while dampening inflammation, thereby accelerating the healing process. RICE quickly became indoctrinated in healthcare settings and society at large; it is still common practice for ice packs or compression bandages to be used immediately after someone sprains an ankle.

Like many theories, however, RICE has not stood up to scientific scrutiny over time. Indeed, rest along with cooling has been specifically shown to have negative consequences for the outcome of the inflammation phase. As W.B. Leadbetter put it: *'Inflammation can occur without healing, but healing cannot occur without inflammation.'*

WHAT DOES 'INFLAMMATION' MEAN?

The Latin origin of the word 'inflammation' is *inflammare*, which means 'set on fire'. It describes the symptoms of the inflammatory process: redness and swelling with heat and pain – *rubor et tumor cum calore et dolore.*

A common misconception is that the swelling following an acute soft tissue injury is synonymous with inflammation. However, the swelling represents the accumulation of waste products produced during the inflammatory process which have not yet been transported away from the site of the injury. This transportation is carried out by the lymphatic system, which is a one-way system where fluid is pumped through lymph vessels back to the heart. This pumping function relies on muscle activity, so actively using muscles is the best way to reduce swelling. Immobilising an injured body part therefore does not contribute to reducing swelling; this inactivity also leads to muscle deconditioning, resulting in a poorer final outcome. And it is not only muscles that suffer due to inactivity. Tendons, ligaments and bones also weaken if they are not regularly stressed, so being completely immobile after an acute soft tissue injury is not something we should do.

Nowadays, we understand that we actually want and need an inflammatory process following an acute soft issue injury, yet at the same time we want to reduce swelling and maintain muscle activity and load. We want to avoid situations that can worsen the injury and we want to avoid the use of anti-inflammatory medications, aka NSAIDs (non-steroidal anti-inflammatory drugs). This development of our understanding over time has led to an evolution from RICE to PRICE to POLICE to MEAT to MOVE*, finally resulting in the latest acronym, **PEACE & LOVE**.

The first part, **PEACE**, applies during the acute phase in the first few days following an injury.

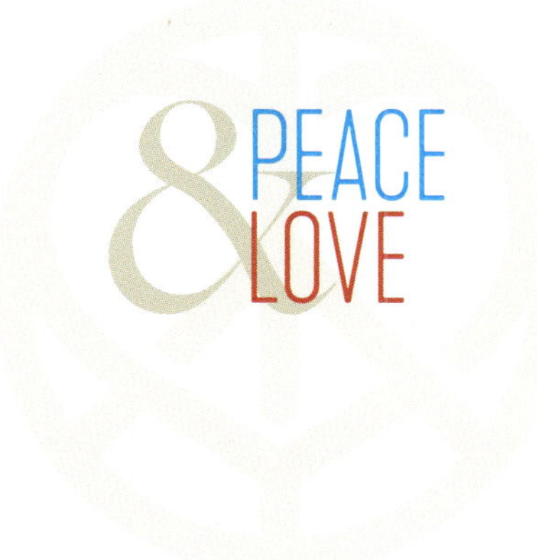

*RICE = Rest Ice Compression Elevation
PRICE = Protection Rest Ice Compression Elevation
POLICE = Protection Optimal Load Ice Compression Elevation
MEAT = Movement Exercise Analgesics Treatment
MOVE = Movement Options Vary Ease

PROTECT

This involves avoiding worsening the injury. If we injure a finger while bouldering, twist an ankle or experience a sudden jerk in a shoulder, it makes sense to end the session early. Although we don't want complete rest for the injured body part, we can limit its use, the load it is under and its range of motion to reduce the risk of worsening the injury. I see that I failed miserably at this first step when I injured my leg in Hueco, although I did switch boulders after the injury.

ELEVATE

Keeping the injured body part above heart level means that fluid accumulated during the inflammation phase can more easily flow back towards the heart via lymphatic system drainage, thus reducing swelling.

AVOID ANTI-INFLAMMATORY MODALITIES

As described on the previous page, we are aiming for a successful inflammatory phase, rather than trying to suppress it. Therefore, we should avoid NSAIDs and cooling measures. Such interventions may reduce pain, which can certainly be desirable in some cases, but they will have no positive effect on the inflammation phase or the final outcome.

COMPRESS

Despite a lack of documentation on the effectiveness of compression bandages, they may help to reduce swelling by providing support around an injured body part. They also appear to be beneficial for quality of life during the period following, for example, an ankle sprain.

EDUCATE

In a world full of internet and YouTube gurus, infinite Google search results, quick fixes and high-tech solutions, it can be difficult to know who to listen to and what information to rely on. Providing good answers related to the type of injury, timescales, prognosis and what a patient can do during the healing process is an important part of a healthcare professional's job, and this is the information we should expect when seeking professional help. The late English physiotherapist Louis Gifford suggested that there are four questions all patients want answered when seeking help:

1. What is wrong with me?
2. How long will it take to get better?
3. What can I (the patient) do?
4. What can you (the healthcare professional) do?

Good answers to these questions, based on the best available knowledge, will give us a quicker start to an active approach to healing and increase our confidence in the process. It will also reduce the need for treatment modalities and medication, while allowing the rehabilitation to progress naturally in the best possible way. Being able to answer all these questions was crucial when it came to handling my own hamstring injury.

While **PEACE** is reserved for the first few days following injury, soft tissue injuries then require **LOVE** in the period following the acute phase.

LOAD

All tissues in the body repair themselves and build up capacity through loading. The underlying mechanism for this is called 'mechanotransduction', and it is now well known how mechanical stimuli increase muscle, tendon and ligament load-bearing capacity. Optimal loading during this phase involves loading the tissue without worsening the symptoms, such as pain or swelling, afterwards.

OPTIMISM

Injuries rarely come at convenient times, and they can negatively affect quality of life and mood. Mental factors such as fear of movement, depression and anxiety can be major obstacles in the rehabilitation process, with a direct negative impact on the final outcome. There isn't necessarily a close relationship between injury severity and symptoms experienced, but there is a much stronger connection between thoughts and emotions and symptoms. It's about how we feel, but also how we handle those feelings. An optimistic mindset leads to better outcomes and prognosis, so we need to focus on the positive in a tough situation. This is one of the reasons why this book has a dedicated section on movement optimism (pages 147–148).

VASCULARISATION

Good fitness isn't necessarily a performance factor for climbers, but after an injury it is important to start general strength and conditioning training early. This increases blood flow throughout the body, potentially reducing pain and improving motivation to continue training. Such forms of exercise also make us feel actively involved in the recovery process; with a finger injury, there is actually a lot of other training we can be doing. Not only does this positively impact the rehabilitation process, but it also makes us stronger and improves our overall physical condition.

EXERCISE

Exercises that target injured tissue structures are the cornerstone of the rehabilitation process. As already explained, exercises provide the specific load to the tissue which optimises healing. Exercises that contribute to regaining strength, full range of motion and confidence in the injured body part are crucial, and should be started as early as symptoms allow.

The most important message you should take away from this section is that **acute soft tissue injuries do not require prolonged periods of rest**. They involve an acute inflammatory phase which is required for optimal healing, but it is then absolutely necessary to load the tissue from an early stage to ensure the best possible outcome. The most common climbing-related injury is an acute pulley rupture in a finger, and the principle of **PEACE & LOVE** applies greatly to this type of injury. Keep this in mind when you read the section on pulley injuries on pages 41–51.

OVERUSE INJURIES

Whereas acute injuries have a clearly defined time of injury (often a specific event), both the cause and the time of onset are less clear in the case of overuse injuries and conditions. Simply put, overuse injuries can be the result of exercising:

TOO MUCH, TOO OFTEN, TOO SOON and with TOO LITTLE REST.

However, it is difficult to be certain about what is too much or too often. Therefore, we consider the load from various perspectives – physiological as well as psychological and social. Let's start with the physiological aspect.

All tissues in the body adapt in response to loading. This is why muscles become larger and can generate more force, why tendons and ligaments become thicker and stiffer, and why bones build more bone tissue. Overall, loading allows us to develop strength and resilience against higher forces. To stimulate this adaptation process, we must expose our bodies to stimuli which they are not already capable of handling. This applies to all types of training – from purely physical, to technical and mental training. If we exceed what the tissues can withstand without then providing sufficient rest so they can adapt, no adaptation will occur; instead, this repeated tissue breakdown may eventually lead to symptomatic tissue damage.

We can use our fingers as an example. By climbing on steeper wall angles and using smaller holds, we can expose our muscles, tendons, ligaments and bones to forces that can make us stronger. This leads to thicker and stiffer pulleys and tendons, thicker bones and broader joint surfaces if we rest adequately between sessions. However, without sufficient recovery, we may experience adverse reactions such as elbow tendinopathy, tenosynovitis within the flexor tendon sheaths and synovitis in the finger joints. In younger climbers who are still growing, excessive loading can cause changes and potentially fractures in the growth plates of their finger bones (read about my own experience of this on page 8). It is difficult to determine exactly where the limit is, but this is the key. If we can control the load, so that there is a balance between stress and recovery, we can both reduce the risk of injury and manage it better if and when it does occur. Rehabilitating an overuse injury is impossible without adjusting the load that caused it; therefore, all rehabilitation programmes should have load management as a fundamental principle.

A good place to start is the **LOVE** protocol (see previous page). Load management is not about a complete unloading, but rather about adjusting the different elements that make up the load. By adjusting both volume (how much we train) and intensity (how hard we train), we can continue training and climbing if we also ensure sufficient rest. Paradoxically enough, loading is a crucial part of managing overuse injuries. In most cases, there are many things we can still train that will have positive effects on our physical and mental well-being. A painful finger may lead us to reduce specific finger training and avoid steep crimping for a short period, but we can still practise technique on larger holds with gentler wall angles, practise clipping techniques while lead climbing, and work on arm strength and basic conditioning.

This way, we provide some reduction in load for the affected finger while simultaneously improving other aspects of our climbing through general training. This general approach to training also has a positive effect on reducing recovery time for an injured finger, and generally has a positive psychological response because we are actively doing something towards getting better.

'IF YOU GO TOO HARD ON YOUR EASY DAYS ... SOON YOU WILL BE GOING TOO EASY ON YOUR HARD DAYS.'

KEIJO HÄKKINEN, WORLD-LEADING RESEARCHER IN POWER TRAINING

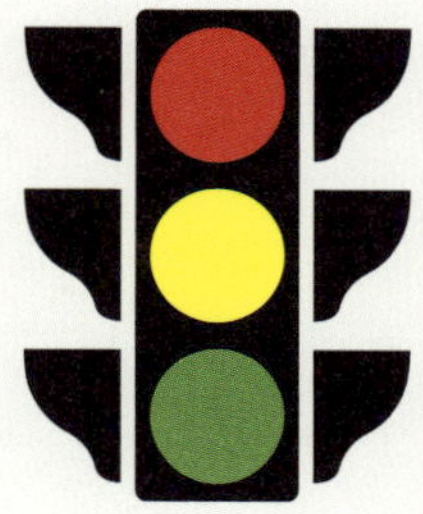

A good method for becoming aware of and monitoring training load over a period of time, such as a week, is labelling sessions as red, yellow or green. Red represents the hardest sessions, green represents the easier sessions, and yellow sessions fall in between. A hard bouldering session for two hours would be considered a red session, and looking back over a week it is possible to see how many red sessions there have been. If there are lots of these sessions within a week, this is not a sustainable training strategy. To improve our climbing ability, we must climb a lot, which means that we must vary our training so it is more sustainable. This could still mean bouldering for two hours, but instead on gentler wall angles, or focusing on technical balance problems. It may not be as physically demanding, but it requires more technical skill.

By combining more general physical training with specific training for an affected body part, we can avoid large fluctuations in the loading rhythm. If a climber is used to climbing and training three times a week but then takes three weeks off completely, there will be a drop in training load. When they start again, they should build up towards their previous level of training load; however, this pattern of peak-drop-peak can contribute to recurring issues. We should strive to maintain a relatively steady workload with only short and moderate fluctuations periodically to vary the load. However, illness, injury, holidays and life in general can cause a drop in training intensity that deconditions us physically. Few of us are diligent enough to gradually rebuild our condition following these periods, and so this often leads to us doing too much, too soon.

Being aware of this can serve as an injury prevention measure: if we incorporate brief sessions of finger and upper-body strength training during times when we have less time or opportunity to climb, we will be much better prepared when we resume climbing again.

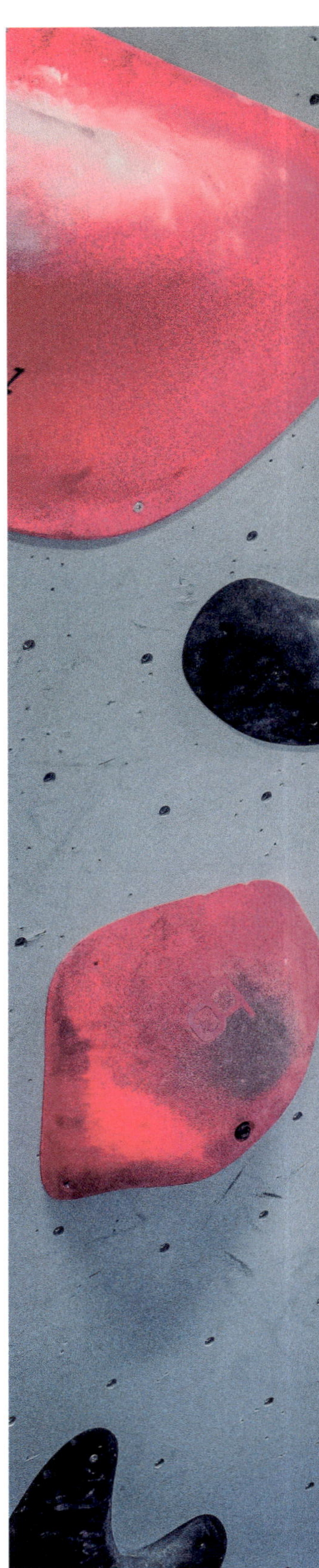

INJURY PREVENTION: MORE THAN JUST TRAINING?

Unfortunately, when we train to become better climbers, injuries and pain are almost inevitable parts of the process. This is why it has been suggested that the term 'injury prevention' is replaced with the term 'risk reduction' – because it is impossible to prevent injuries one hundred per cent. A preventive measure can at best reduce the risk of an injury occurring, but even if we do everything right, there is still an element of chance involved. Bad luck. Shit just happens. Regardless of which term we choose to use, there are steps we can take to reduce our risk of injury, and, if we manage to do the fundamental things well, we have at least done what we can to try to stay injury free.

First and foremost, it is important to distinguish between *external* and *internal* risk factors. External factors are things like whether the safety equipment is in order, whether there are holes in the crash pads or if they are placed next to each other properly so there is no gap which could roll an ankle, whether the last move on a boulder is a sideways dyno, or if your training wall only has small crimps on it. Internal factors concern us as people and how we respond to stressors, and these factors are primarily what I want to highlight in the rest of this chapter.

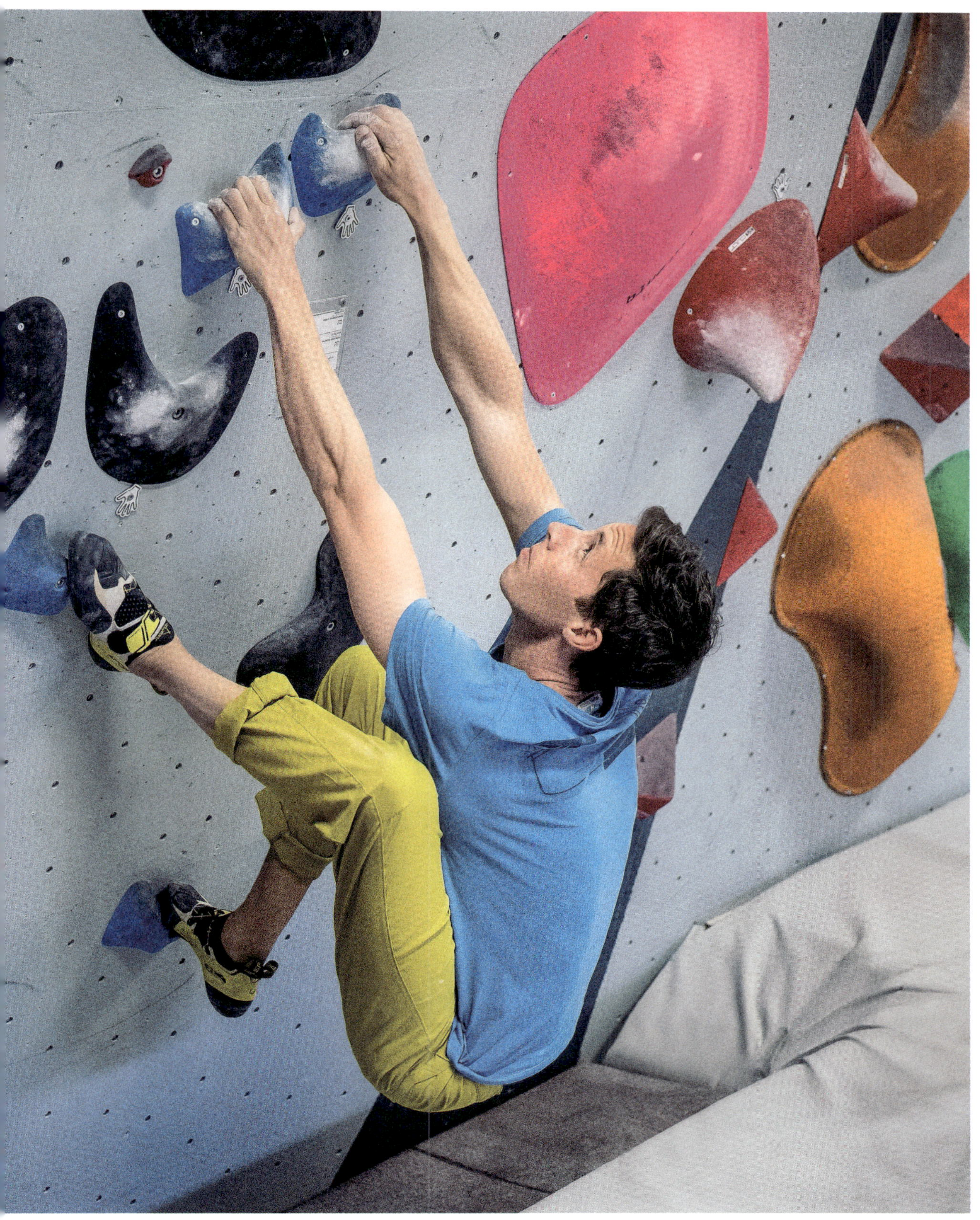

TRAINING LOAD: A PART OF THE WHOLE

Training load is one part of the *total load* we are exposed to, and how much training is too much is very much determined by the individual and depends on several factors. A training process consists of *external load* – volume, intensity, exercise selection and type of training – and *internal load* – how we physiologically respond to the external load and what the outcome is.

This is a simplification of training load, and when we train both hard and frequently, the external training load is generally high. How we respond to this load is influenced by various factors, such as our individual characteristics, training status and age, fitness level, overall physical and mental health status, nutritional status, genetic material and our environment. Therefore, the same external training load can have different outcomes for different people, making it difficult to predict whether a training plan will have the desired effect or if the training load may become excessive. Some parameters are also easier to control than others. For example, it's easier to measure and control deadhangs – hanging motionless from straight arms on a fingerboard – by looking at weight, edge depth and hang time, compared with assessing the load during a climbing session. However, when climbing we can still consider the number of moves per session as an indicator of volume, while wall angle and hold size can be used as indicators of intensity during each session. Many moves on steep walls with small holds will result in a high overall external training load. By reducing volume during such sessions, we can achieve quality workouts at a high intensity, while performing many moves on less steep wall angles with larger holds would result in a session that is higher in volume but lower in intensity. The obvious challenge with climbing is that it's so enjoyable to climb both hard and a lot, that we often end up doing multiple consecutive sessions with consistently high levels of external load.

Several models have been proposed to predict injury risk based on changes in load, the most popular being the Acute: Chronic Workload Ratio (ACWR). This model calculates the training load for the last week (acute training load) and divides it by the average training load for the previous three to six weeks (chronic training load). The greater the difference between these two loads, specifically if the acute training load is higher than the chronic, then the higher the ratio and thus the risk of injury. Although this model quickly gained popularity due to its simplicity, from a scientific perspective it has significant flaws that prevent it from being used as anything more than a measuring tool for external load. There are so many factors other than just the relationship between acute and chronic training loads that contribute to injury risk, that all models are ultimately too simplistic. However, we should still consider the basic principle of managing training load as a risk-reducing measure.

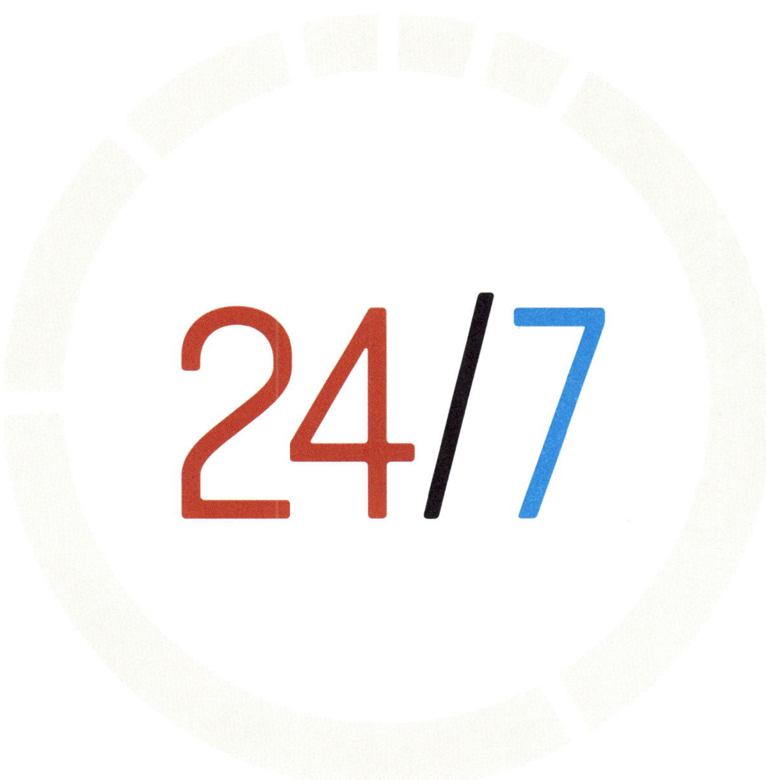

When discussing overuse injuries and load management, we must also consider the concept of *total load*. Unlike training load – which refers to how much and how hard we have trained – total load encompasses *everything* we are exposed to in life, including work, childcare, illness, moving house and so on. There will be periods with intense training, periods with poor sleep quality and periods with increased emotional stress. For example, most parents of young children would agree that this phase in life can be demanding, making it difficult to tolerate the same level of training load as before if they're only sleeping in two-hour intervals while simultaneously working and taking care of a small child or children. Changes in life situations, such as periods of high work pressure or negative relationships, will also increase total load, thereby reducing our capacity to handle additional physical strain. Being aware of how all these elements are interconnected and influence one other gives us an opportunity to adjust our training loads during certain periods, while accepting that it's not always possible to achieve our desired volume.

PHOTO: MARTIN MOBRÅTEN

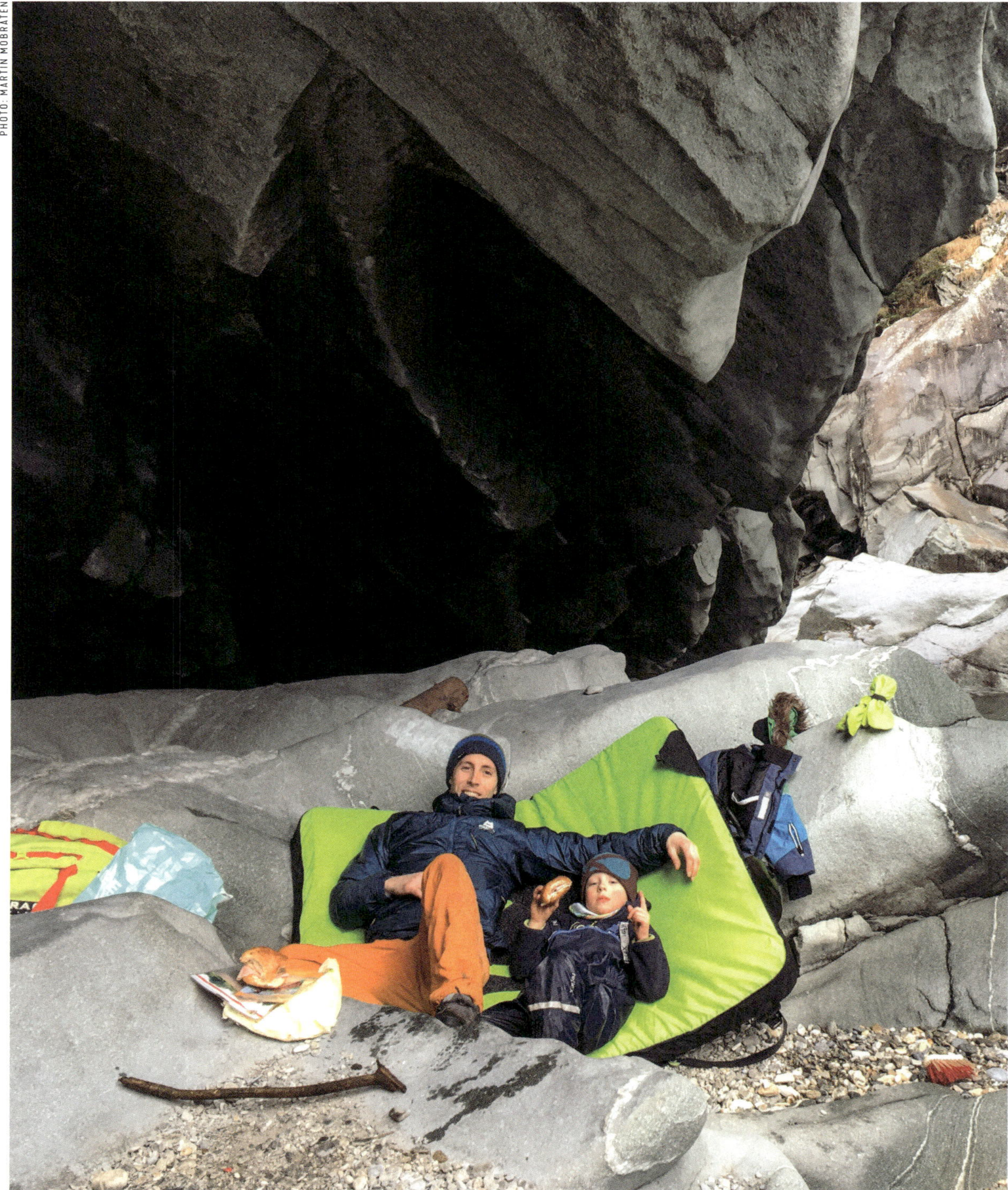

Having children is wonderful, but most parents agree that it can also be exhausting. Periods of reduced sleep affect both training quality and recovery. Considering the wants and needs of another human being affects how we prioritise our own time and makes us think twice about training time and volume. If we're lucky enough to have children who want to join us on a trip, we can also look at it as a long-awaited opportunity to take a slightly longer rest between attempts, so we might be able to complete our project after all! Stian and Kasper (then aged six) enjoying lunch on the pad by Bruno Bloc in Magic Wood, Switzerland.

SOCIAL MEDIA/TV

1 HOUR

TRAVEL TIME

1 HOUR

MEAL TIMES

1 HOUR

FAMILY/FRIENDS

2 HOURS

TOTAL LOAD

TRAINING

3 HOURS

WORK/SCHOOL

8 HOURS

If we have a full-time job and young children and have to squeeze in a few training sessions during the week, our training load may be low, but our total load may be high. The same applies to young climbers/athletes who have to juggle school, friends training and competitions. The total load they're exposed to during the course of a day can quickly end up being very high. A tool that is often used for young athletes is the '24-hour athlete', but I believe it is a useful tool for anyone who wants to structure their training.

The exercise involves looking at our everyday activities and calculating how long each one takes. Sleep, work, school, training, travelling, family, friends and so on. We only have 24 hours at our disposal, so how do we use our time in the best possible way? How do we get the most out of our training sessions? Are we getting enough sleep so that we can recover properly?

SLEEP

8 HOURS

SLEEP AND NUTRITION

Most of us have experienced the effect of poor sleep quality on our bodies, and so it should come as no surprise that insufficient sleep can be a risk factor for sports injuries. Insufficient sleep leads to an increase in physiological demand during physical and cognitive activity, which results in more rapid fatigue compared to if we had slept better and for longer.

Adolescents between the ages of 12 and 18 who sleep for less than eight hours a night are reported to have a significantly higher injury risk compared with their peers who sleep for eight hours or more. Considering that the amount of sleep generally decreases during adolescence, and the risk of sports injuries increases during the same period, we can make an assumption that reduced sleep over time is a risk factor.

Reduced sleep also directly affects how well and how quickly we're able to recover following a training session, thus having consequences for how well we tolerate training load over time. The external load may be the same, but the internal load is significantly higher and will eventually lead to reduced performance and potentially overuse injuries. Additionally, considering that reduced sleep is associated with poorer nutritional status, we now have two important factors negatively affecting our recovery time.

The Norwegian Olympic and Paralympic Committee and Confederation of Sports has developed nutritional guidelines for injury periods (see opposite), but we can also use these guidelines to ensure a nutritional status that can reduce the risk of injuries associated with inadequate nutrition. The most important thing is to have enough energy and carbohydrates available to meet the strain we put on our bodies, and this is particularly important for children and adolescents. A deficit in energy balance is not a sustainable strategy for either adults or youths who want to train extensively, and malnutrition is linked to both physical injuries and mental health problems. A diet consisting of regular meals that include fats, carbohydrates and proteins, as well as the recommended daily doses of fruit and vegetables, is a more than sufficient nutrition strategy for most people to help reduce their risk of injuries.

So, to all of you young and promising athletes – and to all you hard-working parents – **get enough sleep and eat well!**

RECOVERY NUTRITION

EAT ENOUGH FOOD – DON'T LOSE WEIGHT

This is not the time for dieting!

- Important for maintaining muscle mass.
- Protein intake of approximately 1.6–2.5 grams per kilogram of body weight per day.
- Increased energy requirements during and after surgery.

EAT REGULAR MEALS

Breakfast and evening meals are important meals!

Aim for 20–40 grams of protein per meal.

- Regular protein replenishment will stimulate protein synthesis and reduce muscle loss.
- Evening meals should be high in protein.

AVOID NUTRITIONAL DEFICIENCIES

- Check vitamin D and iron status.
- Include antioxidant-rich foods in your diet, such as fruit, berries, vegetables, nuts, etc.
- Increased calcium requirements in the event of fractures and missing periods.

OMEGA 3

2–4 grams per day (two to four capsules per day)

- Increases muscle-building sensitivity in muscles.
- Reduces inflammatory response.

ENOUGH SLEEP, LITTLE ALCOHOL

- Good recovery routines are very important.

NUTRITIONAL ADVICE IN CASE OF INJURY. REPRODUCED WITH PERMISSION OF HEIDI HOLMLUND/NORWEGIAN OLYMPIC SPORT CENTRE.

DIFFERENCES IN AGE AND GENDER

'Everything hurts a little more now. My finger joints ache, my back is stiff and I feel more beaten up after a good climbing session. In my younger years, I could do a one-arm pull-up straight out of bed, but now it feels like my arms are going to snap when I do a pull-up without warming up.'

It is not uncommon for me to hear statements like this at my clinic, or to overhear them at the climbing wall or crag. As we transition from childhood and adolescence into adulthood, through middle age and beyond, there will be differences in how our bodies adapt to different forms of exercise, and recovery times after strength training and high-intensity interval training will vary throughout our lives. There are also differences between genders, further highlighting the fact that we cannot simply use the same training or rehabilitation plan for every individual. When I compare myself as a 40-year-old to myself as a 20-year-old, there is a significant difference in the training volume I can now handle and in how long it takes me to recover; in practice, we see that many people have similar experiences.

However, it is not possible to be definitive about how age alone affects recovery time. The level at which we climb and how long we have been training will influence both the effectiveness of a training plan and our recovery time after a workout. Therefore, it is not necessarily true that a well-trained middle-aged climber recovers significantly more slowly than a 20-year-old beginner.

Knowing oneself and one's own body is crucial for being able to continuously regulate training load through different periods in life.

MENSTRUATION AND INJURIES

Research on this topic is so scarce, that Martínez-Fortuny et al., the authors of the latest major review article in this field, commented: '*The lack of scientific evidence on this topic is remarkable, and further research is needed in order to validate these hypotheses.*' Keeping this in mind, we can still say that variations in hormone production throughout the menstrual cycle are related to increased risk of injury, especially during ovulation.

Factors such as stiffness in connective tissue, neuromuscular control and strength also vary throughout the cycle, and changes in these factors can affect the risk of injury. It is obviously impossible at present to provide specific and general advice on training and injury risk throughout the menstrual cycle, but where an individual is in their cycle can be one of many factors influencing their injury risk.

Athletes are encouraged to monitor their cycle phase and any symptoms, so that they can better adjust their workload during different phases. Having a better understanding of one's own cycle will contribute to making better medical decisions, and being aware of this allows for the adjustment of the intensity and training methods according to what one knows is right for one's body.

The increased openness about training and menstruation is gratifying, because only through more knowledge, improved understanding and better communication among athletes, coaches and healthcare professionals can we optimise health and performance for female athletes.

WARMING UP

In sports that include a structured warm-up programme which targets the specific demands of the sport, it is generally observed that such programmes help reduce the incidence of injuries. This has been demonstrated in sports like football and rugby, and there is reason to believe that it should also apply to climbing. The physiological processes brought about by warming up make muscles, tendons and connective tissues more elastic – thus more resistant to strain, and increase muscle activation, improve coordination and mentally prepare us for activity. For example, it has been shown that 100–130 moves on a climbing wall makes the pulleys more elastic. By performing some portion of this volume on a fingerboard, one can progressively and in control vary grip positions while increasing both load and rate of force development during warm-up, while simultaneously warming up the rest of the body as well.

The goal of our climbing or training session affects the final part of our warm-up. If we are going to have a finger-intensive and hard bouldering session, the last part of our warm-up should include fast pull-ups, jumps to edges and some sets of heavy deadhangs with a 3–5-second hang time. If the focus of the session is more technical, working on elements like balance and weight transfer, the last part of the warm-up should be directed more towards coordination and balance to stimulate body awareness and improve motor-learning outcomes.

SUGGESTED WARM-UP EXERCISES

The aim of the warm-up programme is to get the whole body moving. The exercises presented here can serve as a starting point that you can adapt to your own needs, but I recommend including exercises that involve the upper body and shoulders, hips, legs and of course the arms and fingers. The exercises can be done as a circuit, with the first round easier than round two, so that you gradually increase the load and finish ready to climb.

FLOOR EXERCISES — 10–12 REPETITIONS X2 SETS

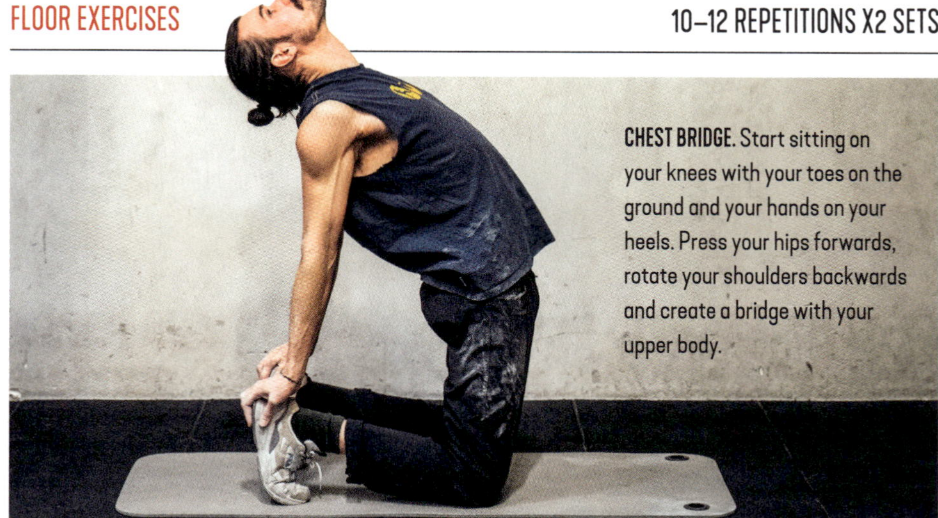

CHEST BRIDGE. Start sitting on your knees with your toes on the ground and your hands on your heels. Press your hips forwards, rotate your shoulders backwards and create a bridge with your upper body.

FLOOR EXERCISES

10–12 REPETITIONS X2 SETS

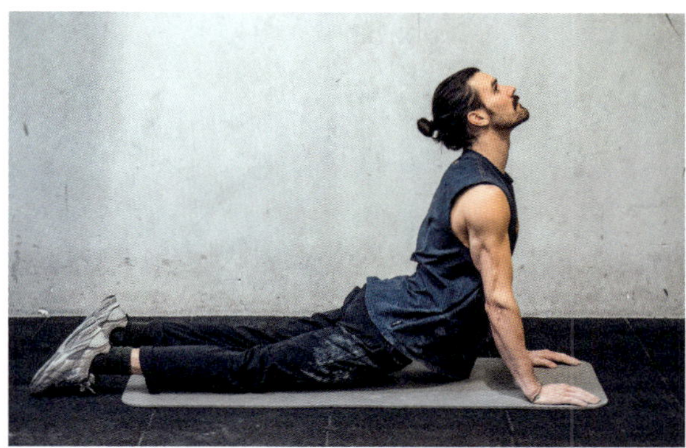

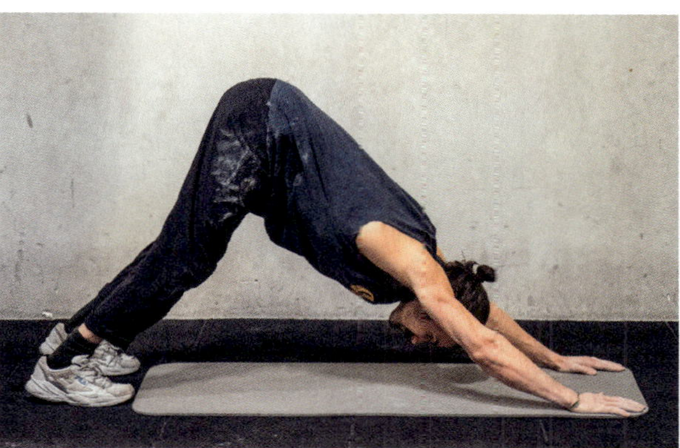

COBRA TO DOWNWARD-FACING DOG. Start lying on your stomach and lift your upper body by straightening your arms. Then push yourself backwards and bring your head and upper body in between straight arms.

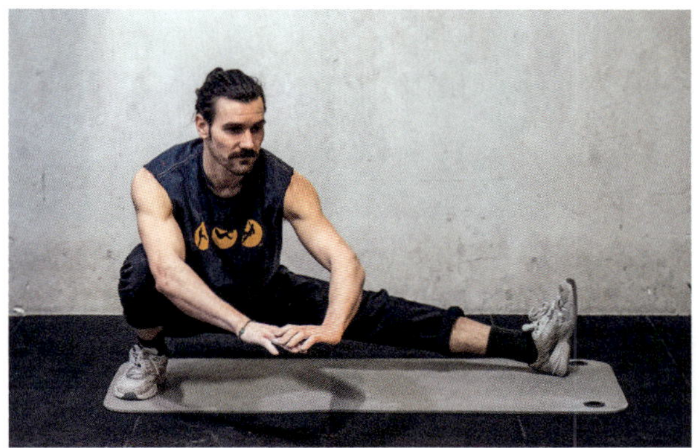

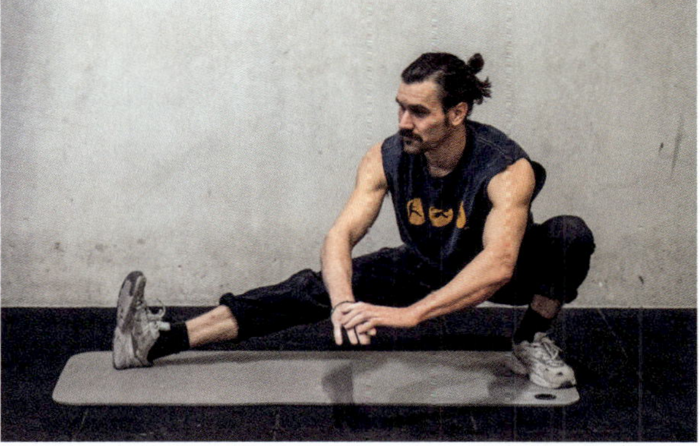

COSSACK SQUAT. Start standing with a wide leg stance. Sit down over one foot while straightening the other leg. Stand up again and do the same on the opposite side.

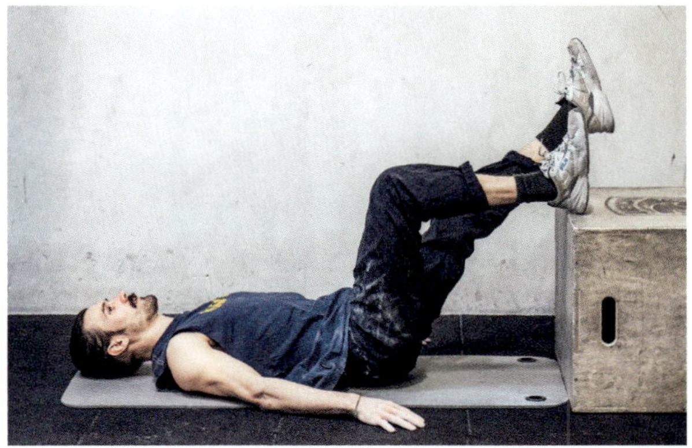

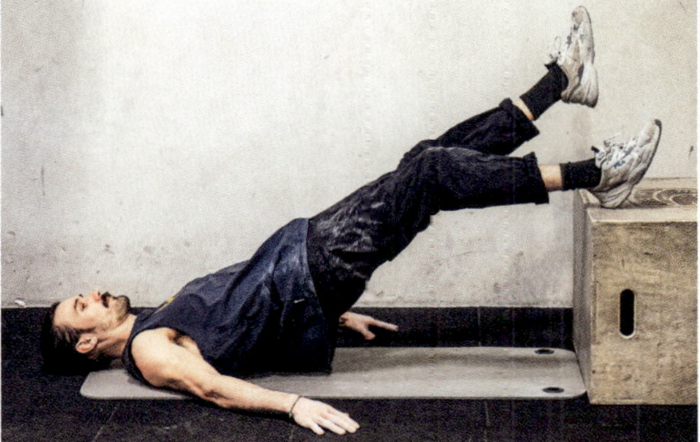

SINGLE-LEG BRIDGE. Start lying on your back with one leg on a box, crash pad or similar. Press your heel against the surface and lift your body off the ground. Vary the angle of your knee and how much you rotate your leg out to the side.

HANGING EXERCISES

5 SECONDS' HANG: 5 SECONDS' REST X5 REPETITIONS X2 SETS

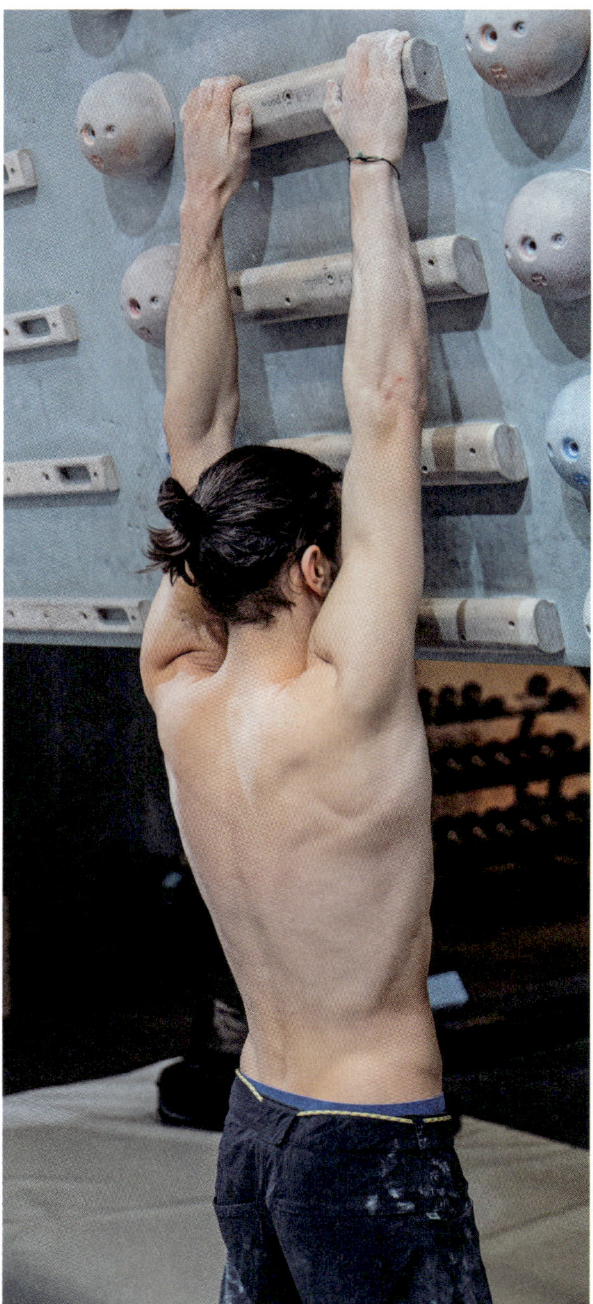

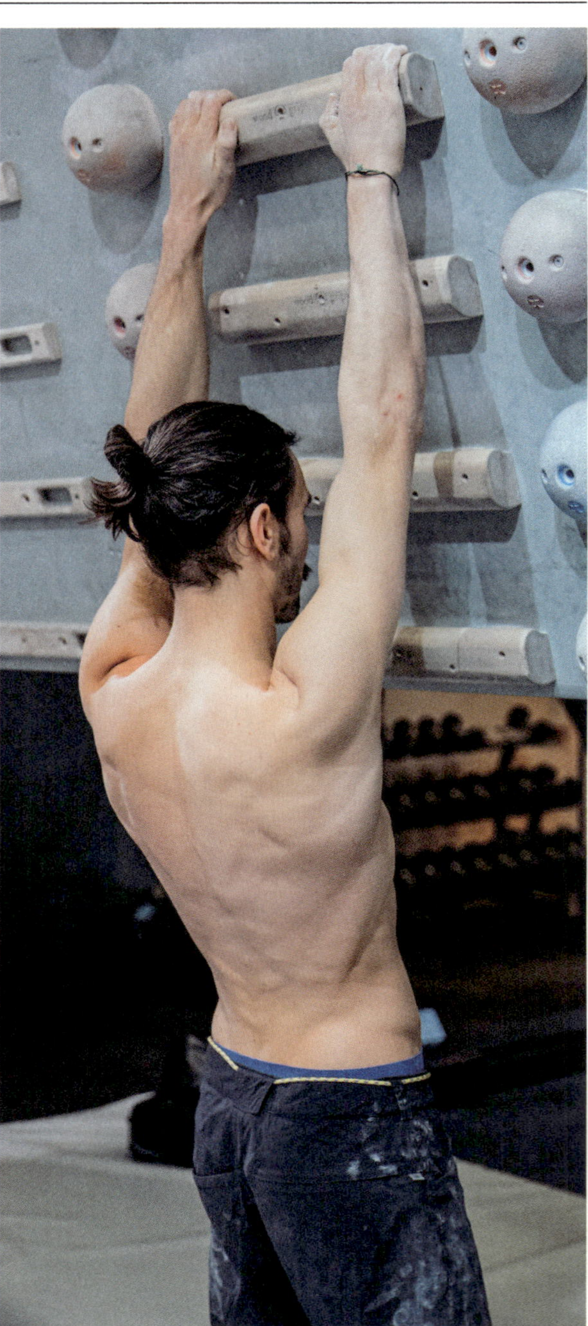

SCAPULAR PULL-UP. Hang passively from good holds. Pull yourself up by pulling your shoulders down and back, keeping your arms straight. Hold the top position for 5 seconds, slowly lower back down, rest for 5 seconds and repeat 5 times.

HANGING EXERCISES

5 SECONDS' HANG: 5 SECONDS' REST X5 REPETITIONS X2 SETS

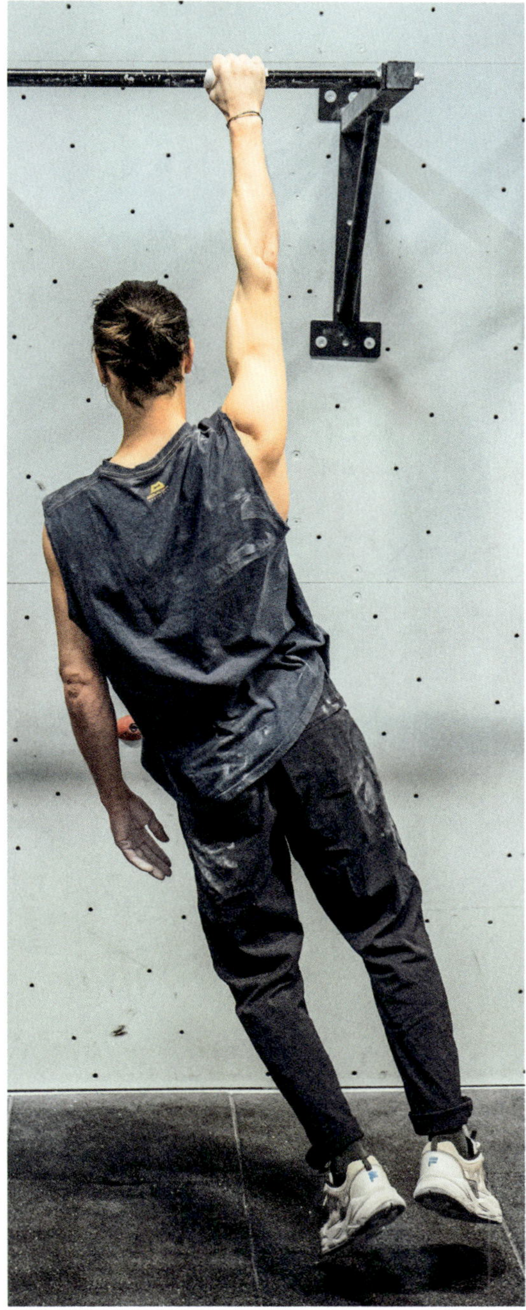

ONE-ARM ACTIVE HANG. Hang from one arm in the top position of a scapular pull-up and hold the position for 5 seconds; repeat 5 times with 5 seconds' rest in between reps.

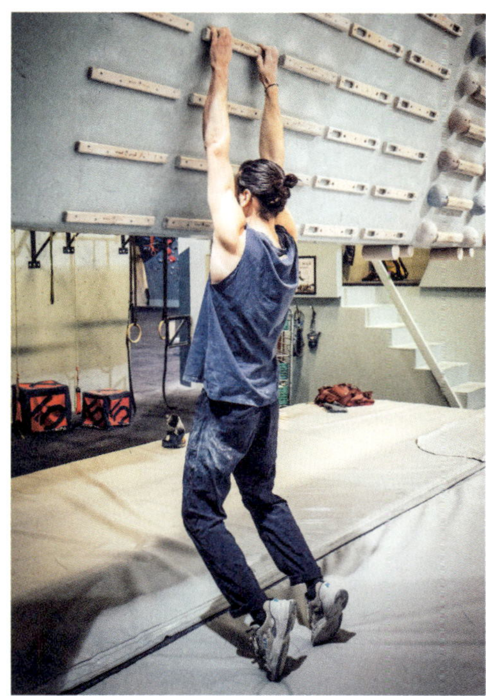

DEADHANG, HALF-CRIMP GRIP. Hang from an edge with a half-crimp grip in the top position of a scapular pull-up for 5 seconds. Rest for 5 seconds, repeat 5 times. Alternatively, if it is too difficult to hang with your full body weight, you can stand on the ground and only take part of your body weight.

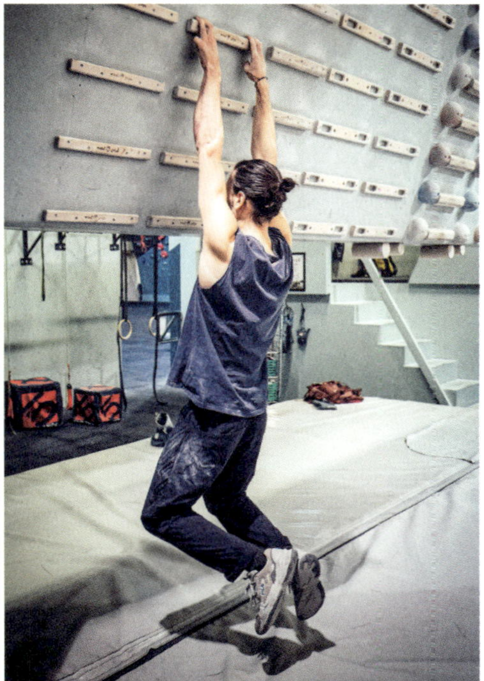

DEADHANG, THREE-FINGER OPEN-HAND GRIP. Hang from an edge with a three-finger open-hand grip in the top position of a scapular pull-up for 5 seconds. Rest for 5 seconds, repeat 5 times. Alternatively, if it is too difficult to hang with your full body weight, you can stand on the ground and only take part of your body weight.

STRENGTH TRAINING

It seems logical that if we become stronger in the areas where the demands are the highest, we will be able to withstand greater forces, thus reducing our risk of injury. From this perspective, all the strength training we do to become stronger climbers, who perform better, can also reduce our risk of injury.

However, here we face a dilemma: if we climb a lot, but at the same time extensively train finger, arm and upper-body strength, we will likely end up with such a high training load that our risk of injury will have increased. But this is a *dosage* problem, not a problem with the training methods themselves. While it's not surprising that self-reported injuries are associated with training facilities such as campus boards, fingerboards and system walls, these are just training installations – they tell us nothing about which training method has been used or at what dosage. An individually tailored strength training programme, aimed at improving finger, arm and upper-body strength while also adapting to the load from other climbing activities, should be a cornerstone in any training regimen – both for performance enhancement, but also as a risk-reduction strategy. By adapting the range of exercises, volume, intensity and frequency, strength training is also a fundamental component in rehabilitation, with the goal of enabling tissues to withstand movement and the stress to which they are subjected.

Therefore, strength training is central to both injury prevention and rehabilitation, where individualisation involves exercise selection and training dose.

Naturally, there is no universal programme, but Glasgow et al. advocate that an optimal loading regime should include the entire neuromuscular system. To accomplish this, strength training should:

1. target the appropriate tissues
2. ensure loading through functional joint range of motion
3. balance compressive, tensile and shear loading
4. vary the magnitude, direction, duration and intensity
5. incorporate neural overload
6. adapt to individual characteristics
7. be functional

If – based on these principles – we regularly train strength over time, research on a wide array of sports has shown that our injury risk can be reduced by up to a third. While climbing-specific research is currently lacking, it is not unreasonable to conclude that climbers can reduce their risk of injury through structured strength training.

PREVIOUS INJURY

The most significant risk factor for sustaining an injury is a previous injury. Some types of injuries, such as strains, tend to flare up again if we don't do a proper job of rehabilitating them. Other types of injuries can predispose us to new injuries in other parts of the body because we modify our technique and movement patterns to compensate, or because pain hampers force development and coordination. A rehabilitation process is therefore not complete until we have worked our way back to – and preferably beyond – the capacity we had before the injury. This also emphasises the need to start loading an injured body part early, and the necessity of taking sufficient time to return to climbing at our desired level. In this regard, the natural variation pattern that climbing provides us with is both a blessing and a curse. A blessing because there is always plenty of climbing we can do, but a curse because there is so much that we can climb, we can climb around the problem instead of addressing it properly. Fortunately, we can use this to our advantage by using climbing as both training and rehabilitation, as long as we are aware of exactly what it is that we are training for.

SUMMARY

Preventing all sports injuries is not possible, but we can influence various factors that collectively can reduce our risk of injury. In climbing, there are many external factors involved, such as checking that all safety equipment is in order, ensuring crash pads are positioned correctly and assessing fall risks. However, there are also many internal factors. I have chosen to highlight the fundamental internal factors associated with increased risk of injury in order to emphasise the message of doing the simple things well and to demonstrate how these factors are closely interconnected. For example, there will be times when we're sleep deprived, times when it's hard to eat both well and enough, and times when it's difficult to train as we'd wished or planned. This is completely okay, but we must make adjustments in our training load during these periods, so that the total load does not become excessive.

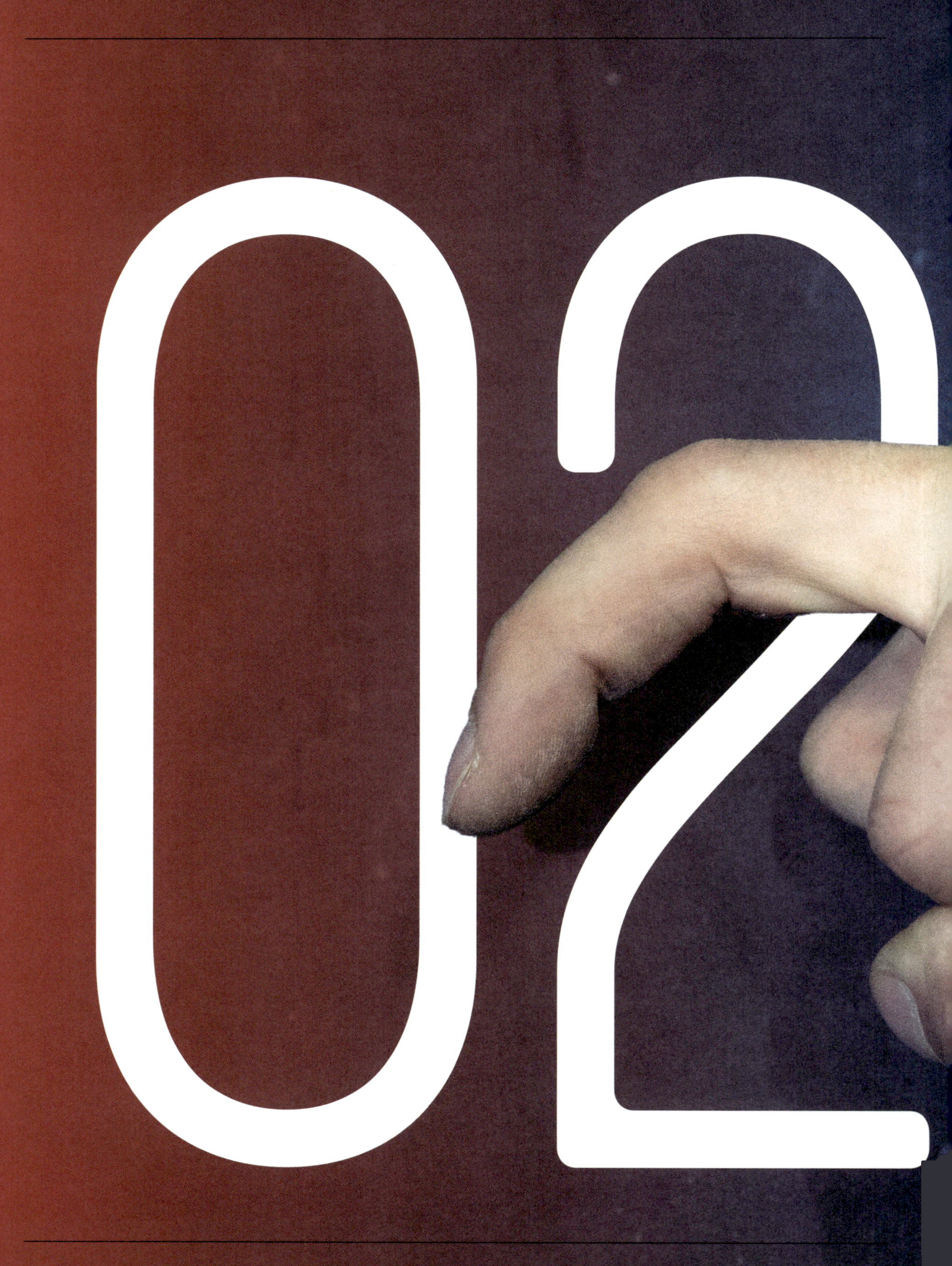
02

THE INJURIES

INJURIES AND BODY PARTS

For each part of the body, the most common injuries and ailments are presented, and for each injury/ailment, the presentation of the injury, diagnosis and management are discussed.

No matter how careful we might be with sleep, nutrition, load management and strength training, injuries are undeniably a part of sports. Even though we can greatly reduce the risk through the measures described in the previous chapter, unfortunately sometimes 'shit just happens'. Just think about the forces our fingers are exposed to when we climb. A large proportion of our body weight is supported on just a few millimetres of grip surface while we move our centre of gravity towards the next hold. The combination of the force development required to maintain a grip position and all the small movements that occur in the finger joints while moving the body can easily exceed what the different structures in the fingers can handle. But this is a risk we take every time we climb. In our pursuit of progress, we will always be balancing on a knife edge between training hard enough and training too much.

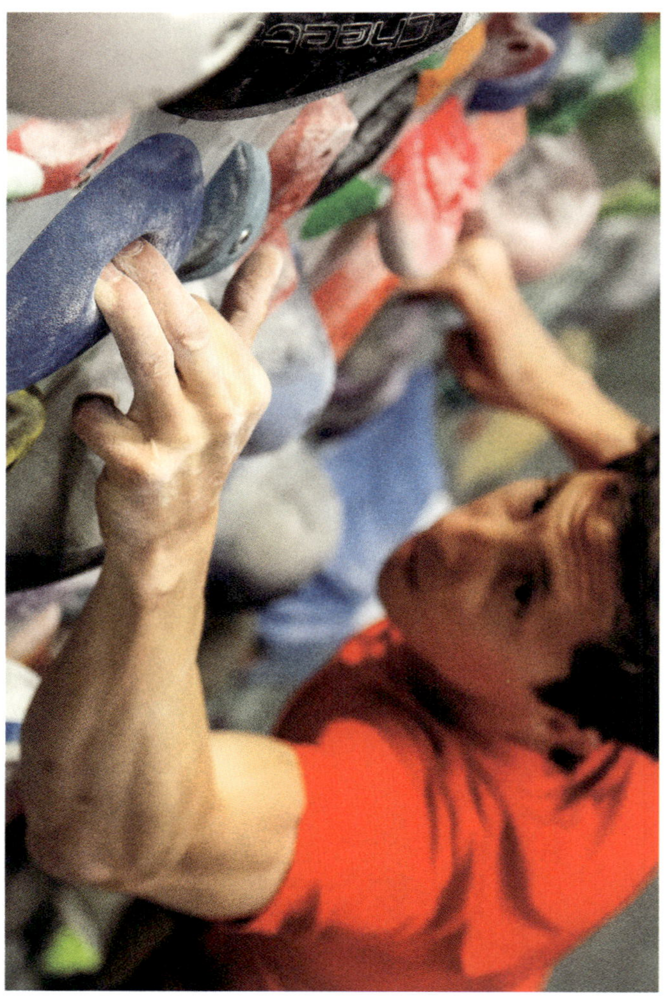

It's important to emphasise that the prognosis – how things will turn out – for the injuries presented in this book is generally good. Most likely, if you pick up one of these injuries, you will fully recover! First and foremost, you need to get an accurate diagnosis so that you can quickly engage in a plan for full recovery. This plan should include specific measures for the injured structure, but also more general ones. After all, a finger injury only concerns one small, albeit very important, body part involved in climbing. Training technique, tactics, and overall strength and conditioning will not only contribute to faster healing, but also make your time off due to injury more fulfilling and help you become a better climber. Remember this as we delve into the dark material regarding the potential injuries that climbers may face.

FINGERS: PULLEY INJURIES

'Pop.' The sound itself is difficult to describe. Perhaps it was more of a feeling? Like something slipping or tearing. But those around me wonder if it was my joint that made the characteristic cracking sound that one can make oneself, so there must have been a sound. I know what this sound means. I've lost count of how many people have described this sound in my clinic. As I stand on the mat and press around my finger where I know the A4 pulley should be, it occurs to me that this doesn't hurt at all. But when I put a little more pressure on my finger, I notice that it's actually quite painful to half crimp, and any remaining hope I have of climbing again today disappears. Inside my head, I've already started forming a plan. A plan for how to get back to doing what I love as quickly as possible. This will be fine. Shit happens. This will be fine.

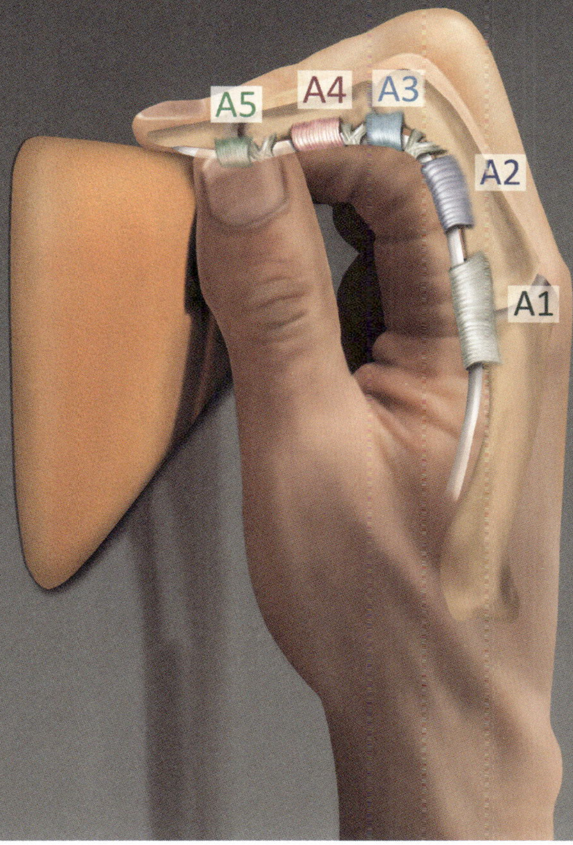

A5

A4

A3

A2

A1

This is my own experience, but it could apply to many others since pulley injuries are by far the most common finger injury in climbing. And the descriptions are quite similar: a palpable and/or audible pop in a finger, followed by varying degrees of pain when pressing on or loading the finger. In the days following the injury, swelling may occur, along with reduced mobility in the finger and decreased strength due to pain during loading.

Each finger has five annular pulleys – except for the thumbs, which have two pulleys each – and they are reinforcements of a larger layer of connective tissue covering the palm and the inside of the fingers. The role of the pulleys is to keep the flexor tendons close against the bones so that the bending of joints becomes possible, much like the rings on a fishing rod allow it to bend.

The finger pulleys are numbered from innermost (A1) to outermost (A5). The stiffest and strongest pulleys are the A2 and A4, and these are also most prone to rupture.

CRIMPING, FRICTION, FORCE AND INJURY

Crimping involves bending the middle (proximal interphalangeal, or PIP) joint of the finger by more than 90 degrees while stretching the outermost (distal interphalangeal, or DIP) joint. The thumb is often placed over the index finger as well. The crimp grip is many climbers' favourite grip position on small holds, yet this hand position is closely associated with pulley injuries – so why do we use it?

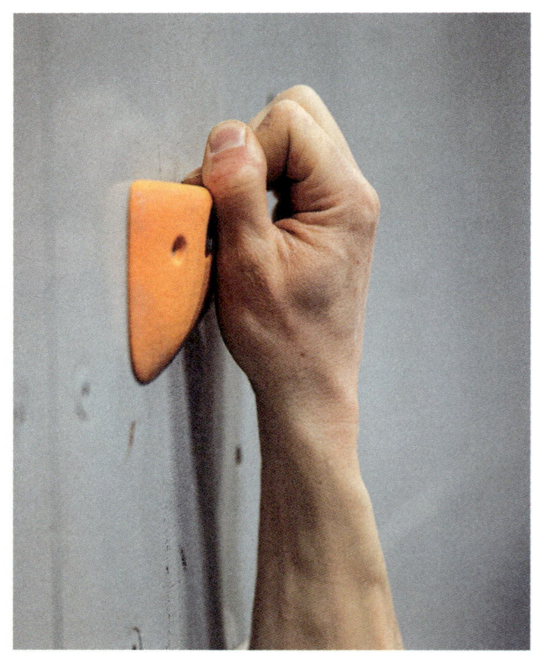

We use it because it offers several advantages:

- we can involve an extra finger (the thumb) to generate force;
- we can move our centre of gravity closer to the next hold when compared with an open-handed grip position;
- and we're improving (lengthening) the lever arm so the flexor muscles can apply more force to the grip surface.

In addition to all of this, the insides of the A2 pulleys are lined with small grooves that match the surfaces of the superficial flexor tendons. This allows the surfaces to lock against each other, like a Chinese finger trap, when the friction between the structures increases. Due to how these grooves are organised in relation to one other, tendons can slide relatively unhindered inwards – when the fingers bend – but encounter resistance outwards, both during static holds and when fingers straighten under load. This locking mechanism – called *tendon locking mechanism* – is what allows bats, birds and certain climbing mammals to hang from their fingers and toes without using muscle power to maintain grip.

By measuring differences in force development when actively trying to flex fingers against resistance versus hanging still, we see that this system can bear more weight while hanging. The difference lies in the friction created between tendons and pulleys. Single studies have shown that friction accounts for up to nine per cent of force development at mid-joint level in a finger. This means that by crimping while hanging, either nine per cent less muscular effort is required, or nine per cent more force can be exerted on a hold during maximum muscular work. Friction between tendons and pulleys is believed to play a role in pulley injuries since these injuries often occur due to a sudden increase in load that causes the fingers to straighten slightly – eccentric loading – thereby increasing the degree of friction.

The tendon locking mechanism also directly affects how we should train finger strength. To influence pulleys so they can withstand higher loads, it is actually beneficial to train a controlled crimp grip. On a fingerboard, we can easily adjust both weight and duration while being certain that unexpected increases in load should not occur. This training will over time lead to thicker and stiffer pulleys, and will also reinforce the correct use of the crimp grip position. And this is important because when climbing on small holds close to our maximum level, we'll almost certainly need to crimp.

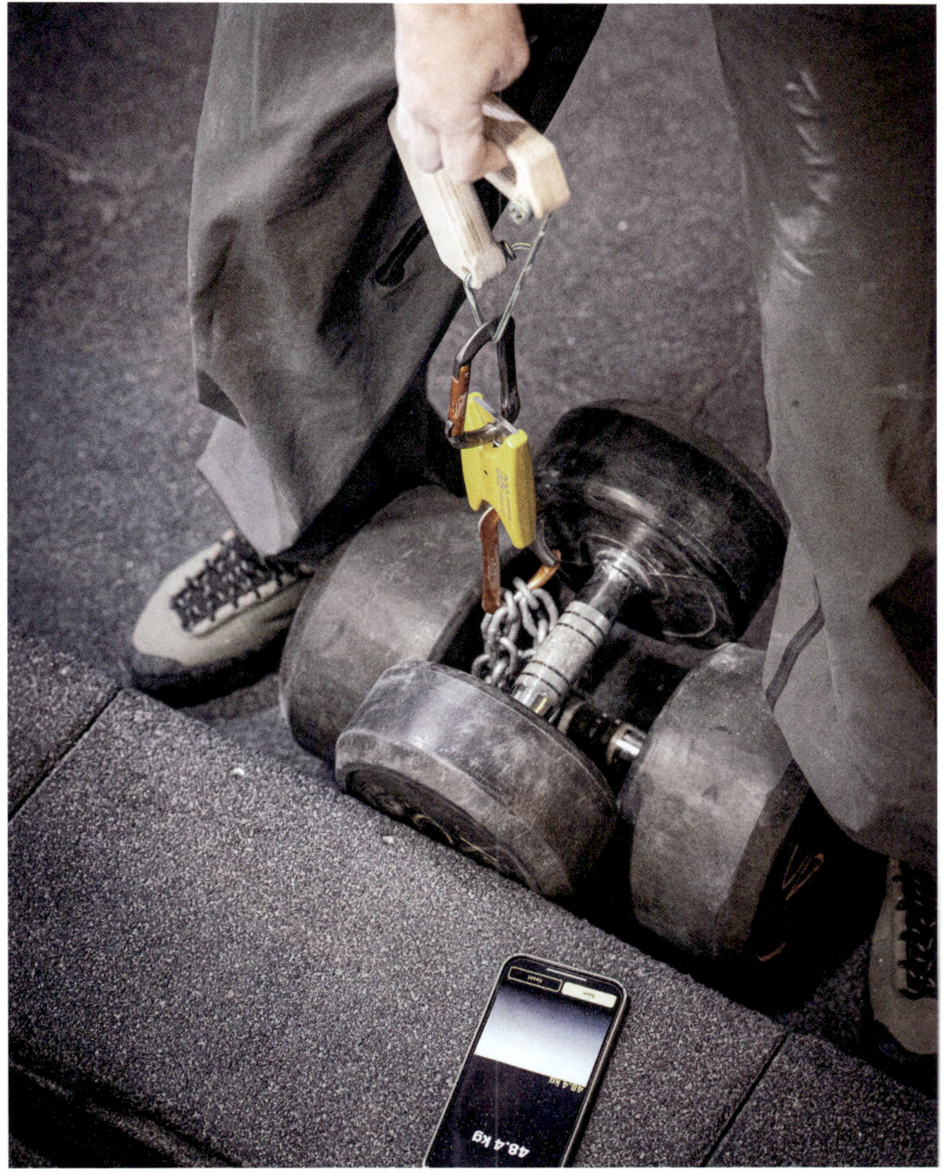

By using a grip tool and a load cell (such as a Tindeq) fixed to the ground, we can accurately measure how much force we are able to produce by curling our fingers against the grip. There is no movement, so the muscle contraction is isometric, but the load cell registers how much force we are able to produce against solid resistance, without the extra help we get from the locking mechanism in the connective tissues.

On the other hand, we try to avoid using the locking mechanism for optimal muscular effect during training. The method of *overcoming isometrics* has been used in strength training for several years, but it is only recently that climbers have realised its potential. With portable force sensors/cells and fingerboards, it's easy for us to curl our fingers against fixed resistance and accurately measure force development (see photo above). A less technological variant involves performing similar movements with our fingers on a fingerboard while standing on bathroom scales and seeing how many kilograms we can subtract from our body weight. Since we avoid the locking mechanism in both cases, we can train to increase our finger strength without putting too much strain on the connective tissues.

MECHANISM OF INJURY AND DIAGNOSIS

When a finger is bent, the flexor tendon is pushed against the pulley system. If the load becomes too great, the pulley may rupture partially or completely – referred to as partial and total ruptures. In unfortunate cases, multiple pulleys can rupture simultaneously, known as multiple ruptures.

The most common ruptures are to either the A2 or A4 pulleys, and they are most often caused by a combination of small hold, crimp grip and a sudden increase in load. For example, this could happen if a foot slips while you are crimping hard, or while you are transitioning from an open-hand grip to a crimp grip. Rupturing a pulley sounds and feels more dramatic than it actually is. In many cases, there may be an audible 'pop' when the pulley ruptures, followed by pain upon loading of the affected finger. Swelling will gradually occur around the torn pulley, causing stiffness when bending the affected finger.

It is advisable to have an examination to confirm that it is indeed a pulley injury and to assess its extent. In most cases, a clinical examination supplemented with ultrasound imaging should suffice.

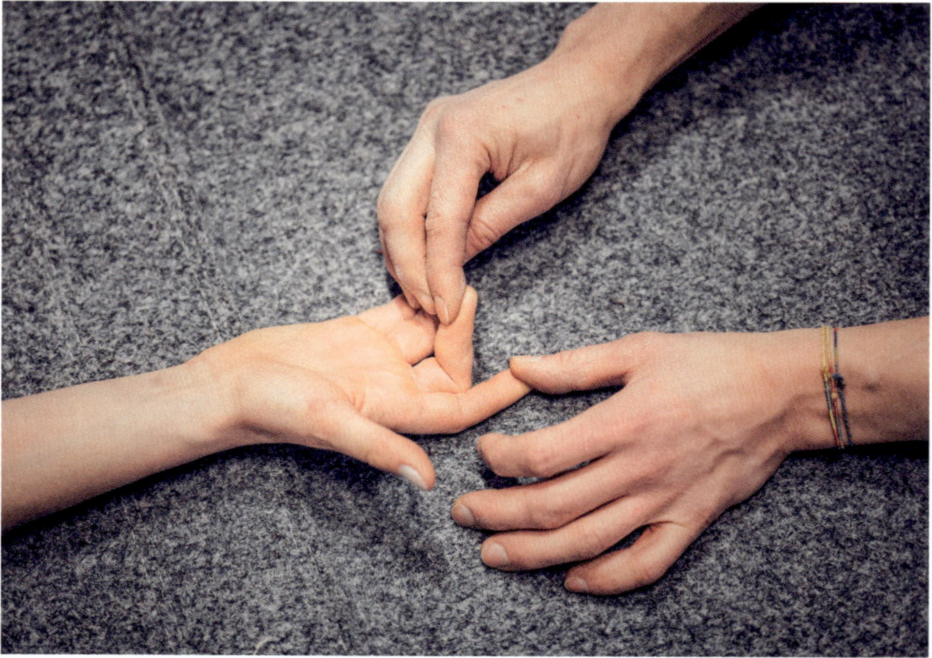

Lay your hand flat with your palm facing up. Bend at the middle joint – the PIP joint – and press the fingertip against resistance, such as another finger. Pain over the A2 or A4 when the finger is stressed in this way may indicate a pulley injury, but this should also be consistent with an acute event that triggered the injury.

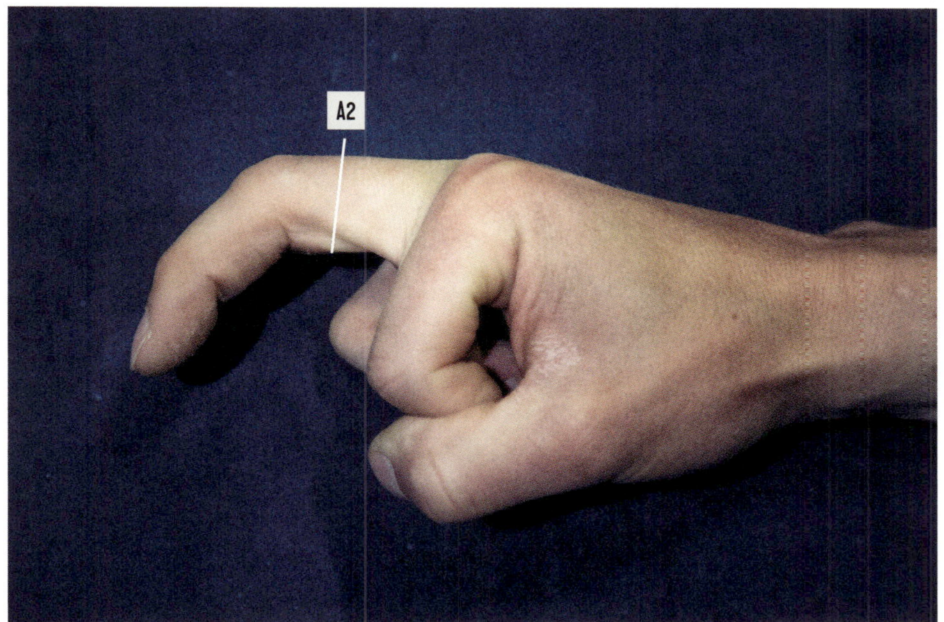

MANAGEMENT

Even in larger injuries involving two or three pulleys, the focus is on rehabilitation, but it is important to determine the extent of the injury in order to tailor this rehabilitation as best as possible. German doctor and climber Volker Schöffl has proposed a classification and rehabilitation protocol for different types of pulley injuries, but, in my opinion, this is relatively conservative and there are significant individual differences in how quickly you can progress with rehabilitation. For example, an A2 rupture may require a slightly slower progression than an A4 rupture, and two climbers with A2 ruptures may also have unique rehabilitation processes. Currently, no one has the definitive answer to how to rehabilitate pulley injuries optimally. The key questions revolve around how soon we start loading and how quickly we proceed with different types of loads.

Once a pulley injury has been diagnosed, it is appropriate to give the affected finger a few days of rest. However, rest does not mean keeping it completely still; it is important to move the finger even if you do not exert much strain on it. Although the ligament itself will not heal back to its original form because of the formation of scar tissue, it is important to create tension in this scar tissue so that it shapes itself as best as possible for future load bearing. In cases of multiple ruptures, however, using a splint – a so-called pulley ring – is important for stabilising the flexor tendons against the bones. This way, over time, scar tissue will adhere more closely to the bones and take over the

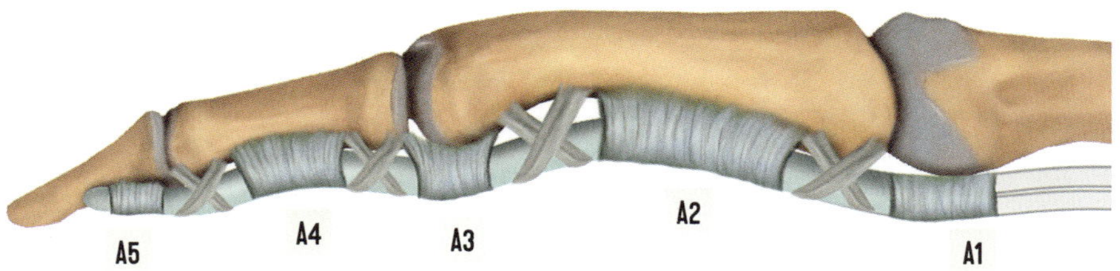

function that was previously performed by the pulleys. As mentioned earlier, pulleys enable the bending of finger joints; if tendons are not held against bones and instead bowstring from the palm to fingertip, this will result in loss of function while also leading to clawing fingers.

The use of pulley rings is also recommended for total A2 ruptures based on the same principle of stabilising the tendon against the bones. However, only one study has been conducted on this approach, and although the results were good, they have not been compared to a control group that did not use a splint. Therefore, it is difficult to say whether this approach is better than not using a splint and whether it is necessary for achieving good short- and long-term outcomes. It is important to note that isolated A2 ruptures have only recently been treated with splints, and we know that this injury has a good prognosis without negative long-term effects even without using a splint.

Whether a pulley ring is used in the first few weeks before loading or if loading is started early on, the injured finger must be loaded. As mentioned earlier, it is through loading that scar tissue settles down in the best possible way and provides both tendons and connective tissues with the elasticity, stiffness and capacity needed for climbing again at your desired level. Naturally, this load also increases the muscular force development you are completely dependent on. By using fingerboards or grip tools with weights or force sensors/cells, you can maintain control over weight, time under tension, grip position and tempo.

Loading an injured finger will eventually cause pain, but as long as it's not so painful that it becomes impossible to handle, you can challenge it. The most important thing is realising that rehabilitating an injured finger cannot be achieved by training pain free, and the pain felt during training is not dangerous. If you load too heavily, you won't be able to generate any power because it will hurt too much, resulting in ineffective training. If you progress too quickly, you may experience increased swelling after training which is also counterproductive as it disrupts continuity in training. Therefore, you must aim to find a 'sweet spot' between load and symptom response, focusing primarily on potential increased swelling after training. The first priority is to gradually increase the load, and you should usually start with open grip positions on relatively good holds (>20-millimetre-deep grip surface) before gradually progressing to half-crimp grips and smaller holds. When the pain reaches a point where increasing weight becomes impossible, you can make the

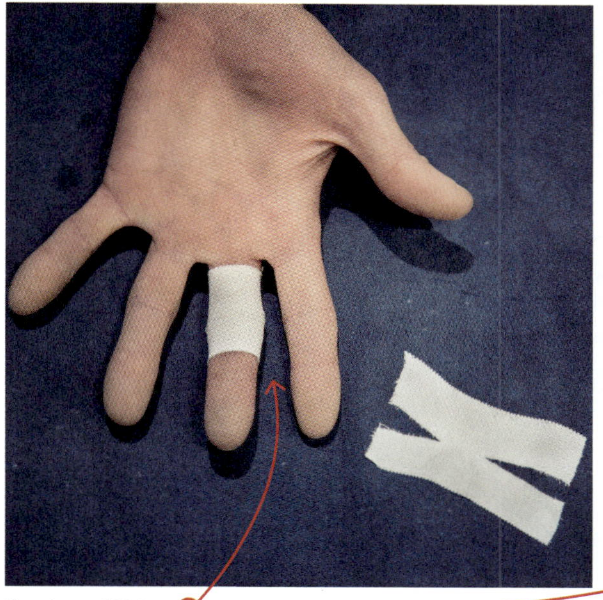
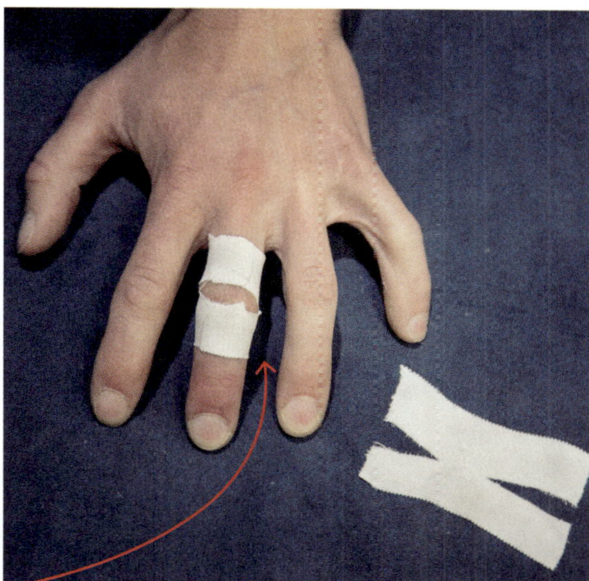

H-taping an A2 injury.

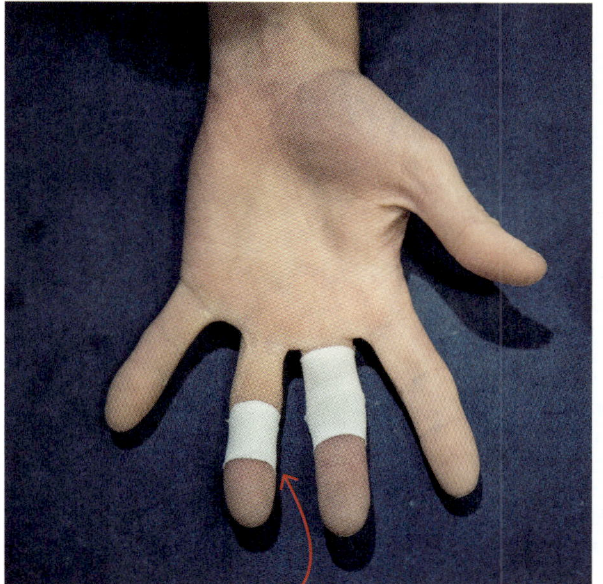
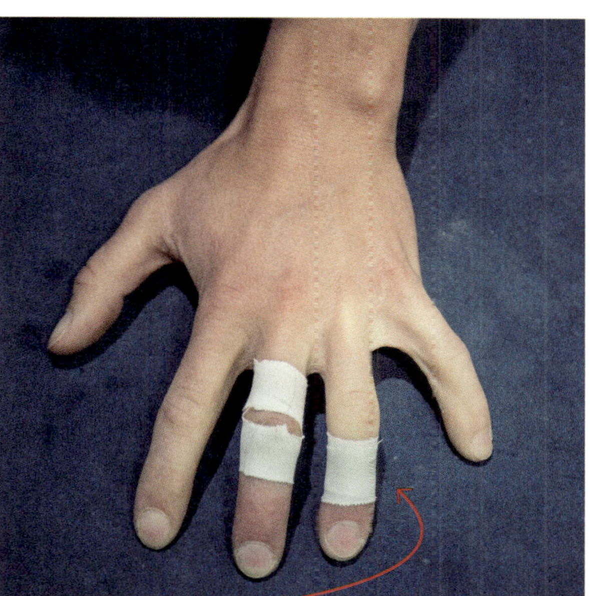

Circular taping an A4 injury.

In the first few months after a pulley injury, it is recommended that the finger is taped to relieve stress. H-taping is recommended for A2 injuries (see photos, top left and top right) and circular taping is recommended for A4 injuries (see photos, bottom left and bottom right). The tape should be applied tightly to provide the best possible support, but be careful to maintain blood flow to the finger. As you gradually put more load through the finger, the tape will no longer have the same supportive function and there is no need to tape a previous pulley injury once you have returned to full weight bearing.

training more challenging by increasing hang time to fatigue the muscles. However, it is important to be able to increase load during rehabilitation, and as load increases, hang time decreases.

During rehabilitation, climbing is important for maintaining movement skills, and initially, it will be crucial to control movements and grip positions on the wall. As you feel confident in increasing load in the specific training, you can also challenge yourself more on the wall, but here the focus should still be on experiencing progress with the finger rather than being able to complete a boulder problem or route. You should gradually work towards developing as much force with the injured finger as before the injury, and this will involve being able to develop this force quickly. This can be done through jump-starting or kick-starting to campus rungs or different holds, where the key is to hold the position on the grip or hold you have jumped to. For example, you can start with a short distance – i.e. less speed in the movement – on good campus board rungs, and then progress to increasing the distance, using smaller holds and different hold types on various wall angles.

This progression ladder – starting with as much weight as you can tolerate and slightly longer hang times, then increasing the weight and reducing hang time, and finally working on rate of force development – will enable you to gradually return to your previous level. And there is no reason to stop there. By continuing this training, you will gradually become stronger than before the injury, thus turning a period of injury into something positive.

There is no definitive answer as to how long the process will take before you are back at your previous level, and from experience I have seen significant individual differences. However, from a purely biological perspective, it makes sense to estimate 8 to 12 weeks before the tissue allows for a load that approaches where you were before the injury. Another crucial factor is how confident you are when loading the finger. Some people have no problems with this, while others are naturally more reserved. This adds another dimension to rehabilitation. It's not just about loading in order for the tissue to withstand stress, but also about loading in different ways to regain confidence in pushing yourself as much as possible. The time it takes for this can vary greatly, but from experience many people are physically and mentally ready to return to their previous level three to four months after an A2 pulley injury.

And if you do rupture a pulley ... don't worry! There is nothing about an A2 pulley injury that suggests you won't reach your desired climbing level.

SUGGESTED REHABILITATION: **PHASE 1**

Load the tissue early in a controlled way.
Avoid an increase in pain and swelling during and after training. As the pain subsides, you can load heavier; if there is no subsequent swelling, you can move on to subsequent phases.

GRIP POSITION:
Four-finger half crimp on a 20mm edge and/or an open grip position on a sloping edge.

METHOD:
No-hang on a fingerboard or with a grip tool, adding weight or using a load cell.

DOSAGE:
15 seconds' hang time with an acceptable level of pain; 5 sets performed daily.

CLIMBING:
On shallower wall angles (<30 degrees), using open grip positions. Focus on footwork, balance, weight transfer and clipping technique.

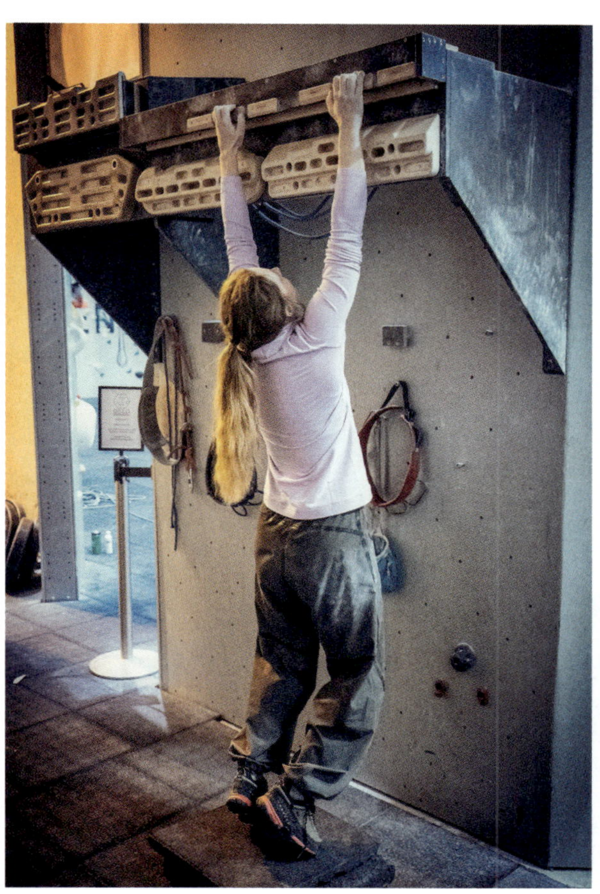

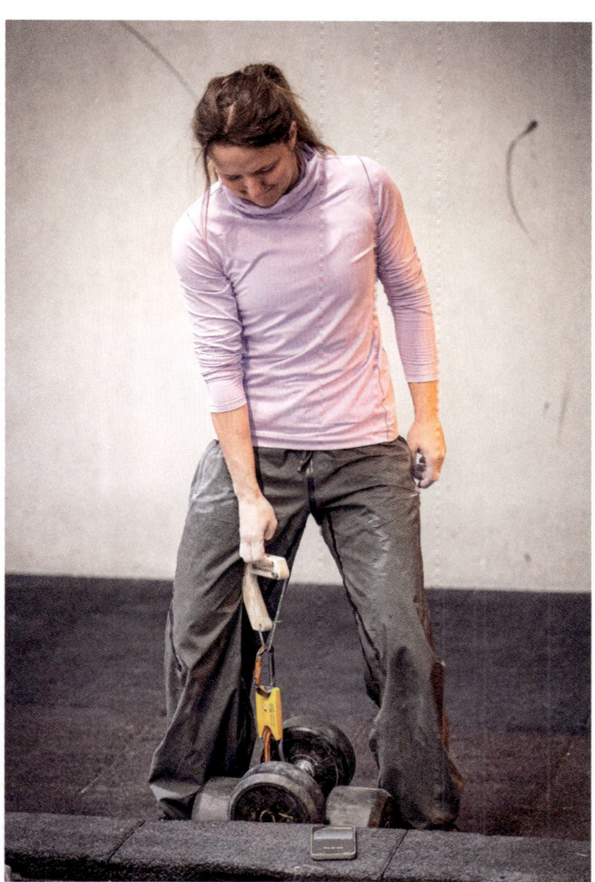

NO-HANG

By standing on the floor and pressing your fingertips against a hold/grip tool (such as a fingerboard), you can load the injured finger with as much weight as you can tolerate in terms of pain. This is a simple and low-tech way to get started with weight bearing, but it will not show you how much you can actually load the finger. You could therefore stand on bathroom scales and see how many kilos you can take off your body weight.

LOAD CELL

The best way to load a finger is to use a grip tool with a load cell and perform 'overcoming isometrics' as explained on page 43. This will give you an accurate measure of how much force you can develop before it becomes too painful to continue. In this way, you can measure progress in terms of increased strength development and manage progress according to symptom response during and after training.

SUGGESTED REHABILITATION: **PHASE 2**

Gradual increase in load on a fingerboard or with a grip tool.

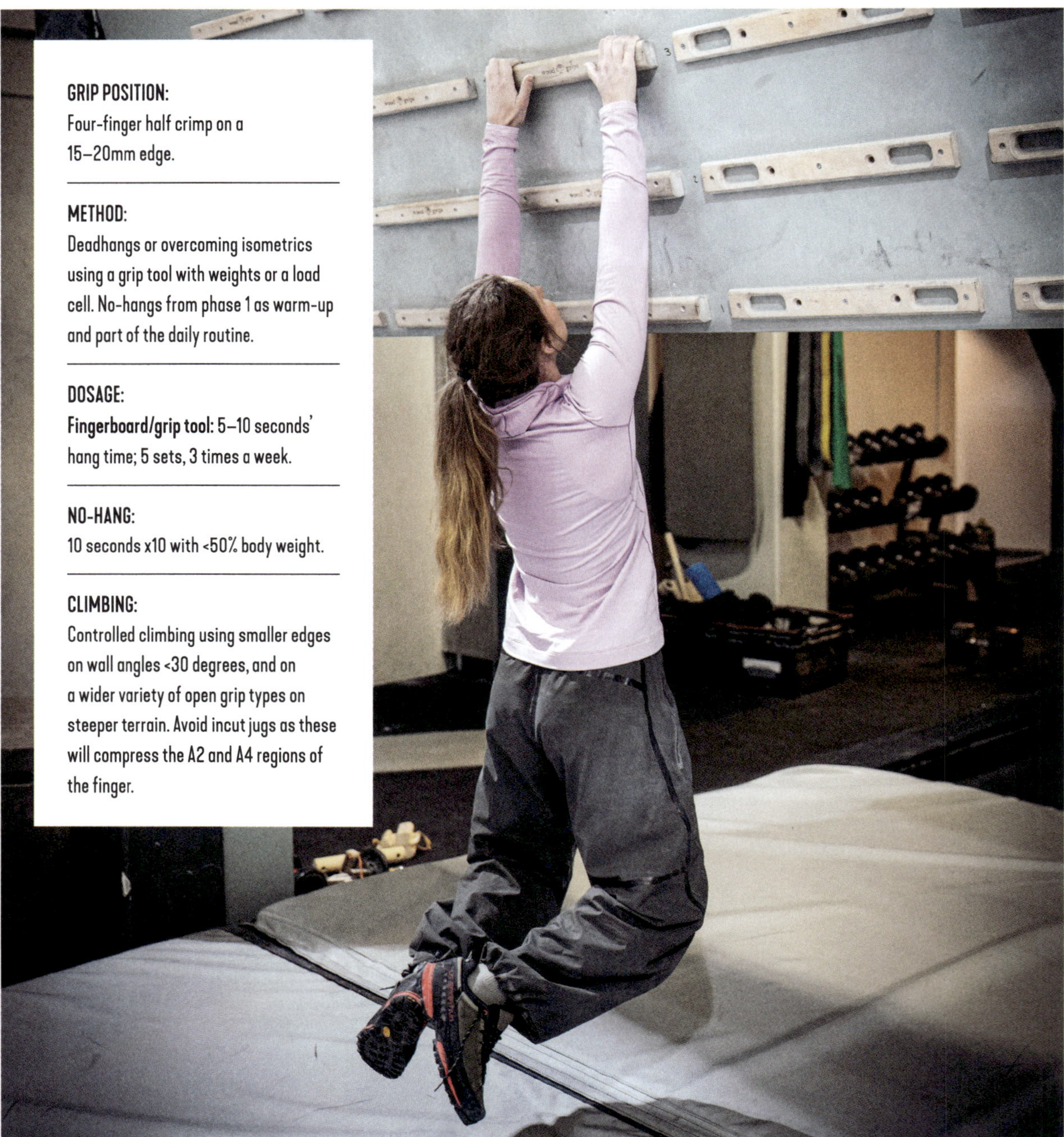

GRIP POSITION:
Four-finger half crimp on a 15–20mm edge.

METHOD:
Deadhangs or overcoming isometrics using a grip tool with weights or a load cell. No-hangs from phase 1 as warm-up and part of the daily routine.

DOSAGE:
Fingerboard/grip tool: 5–10 seconds' hang time; 5 sets, 3 times a week.

NO-HANG:
10 seconds x10 with <50% body weight.

CLIMBING:
Controlled climbing using smaller edges on wall angles <30 degrees, and on a wider variety of open grip types on steeper terrain. Avoid incut jugs as these will compress the A2 and A4 regions of the finger.

DEADHANGING

In this phase you can introduce hanging exercises in addition to continuing the training from the previous phase. Start with relatively good holds and lift your legs off the floor so that you can hang freely from your fingers.

SUGGESTED REHABILITATION: **PHASE 3**

Increased weight, increased rate of force development and increased demands on the finger during climbing.

GRIP POSITION:
Half crimp on a 6–20mm edge. Full crimp during no-hangs to re-introduce the grip position in a controlled way.

METHOD:
Deadhangs or overcoming isometrics using a grip tool with weights or a load cell. No-hangs from phase 1 as warm-up and part of the daily routine. Kick-start/jump-start to a variety of grip types, gradually increasing distance and reducing hold size.

DOSAGE:
Deadhangs/grip tool: 3–5 seconds' hang time, focusing on rate of force development. Perform as repeaters: 3–5 seconds' hang time x4 with 5 seconds' rest between reps; 4 sets, twice a week.
Consider the need for daily no-hangs.

KICK-START/ JUMP-START:
4 jumps;
2–3 sets, 2–4 times a week.

CLIMBING:
Specific training on smaller edges on steeper terrain, working on single moves to and from half-crimp and full-crimp grips.

An acceptable level of pain that does not hinder force development while loading is okay. Worsening of pain during exercise indicates excessive load. Increased swelling the following day is also a response to excessive load. The basic principle is frequent short sessions, with gradually increasing load and decreasing hold depth.

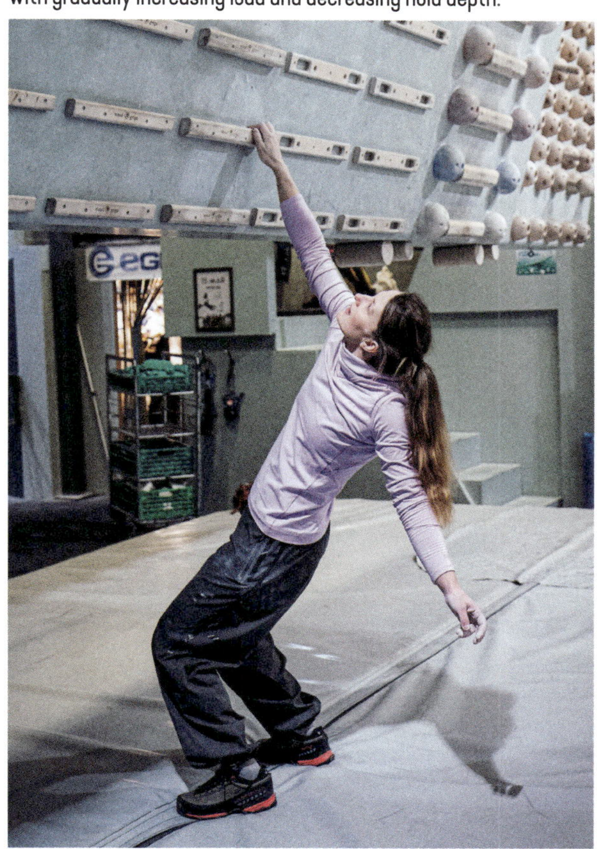

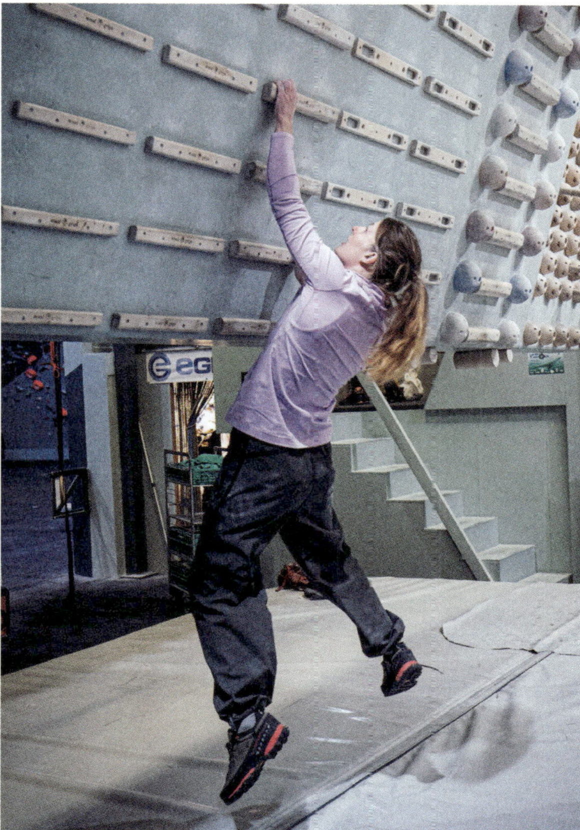

JUMP-START
By introducing jump-starts into rehab, you can stimulate rate of force development for the flexor muscles of the fingers and increased stiffness in the connective tissues. This is often perceived as scary following a pulley injury, so this exercise is a good way to build confidence in latching a hold in the half-crimp grip.

FINGERS: TENOSYNOVITIS

'I wonder if I've ruptured my pulley. It hurts here, where I've read the A2 pulley is, but I can't remember an acute incident and I didn't hear or feel anything pop in my finger. Now the finger is swollen, it hurts to crimp and it hurts to press directly on the area.'

The flexor tendons of the fingers lie inside a tendon sheath, which creates a tunnel through which the tendons can slide friction-free. The tendon sheath consists of a membrane – which is called the synovial membrane – and a stronger fibrous layer above this. The synovial membrane produces synovial fluid, and, together with the annular pulleys, this complex holds the tendons close to the finger bones and provides them with nourishment. In cases of irritation or inflammation of the synovial membrane, the production of synovial fluid increases, leading to swelling within the tendon sheath. This is called *tenosynovitis*, and it is one of the most common conditions I see in clinical practice with climbers. The condition results in a swollen finger that is painful to load and touch, and sometimes one

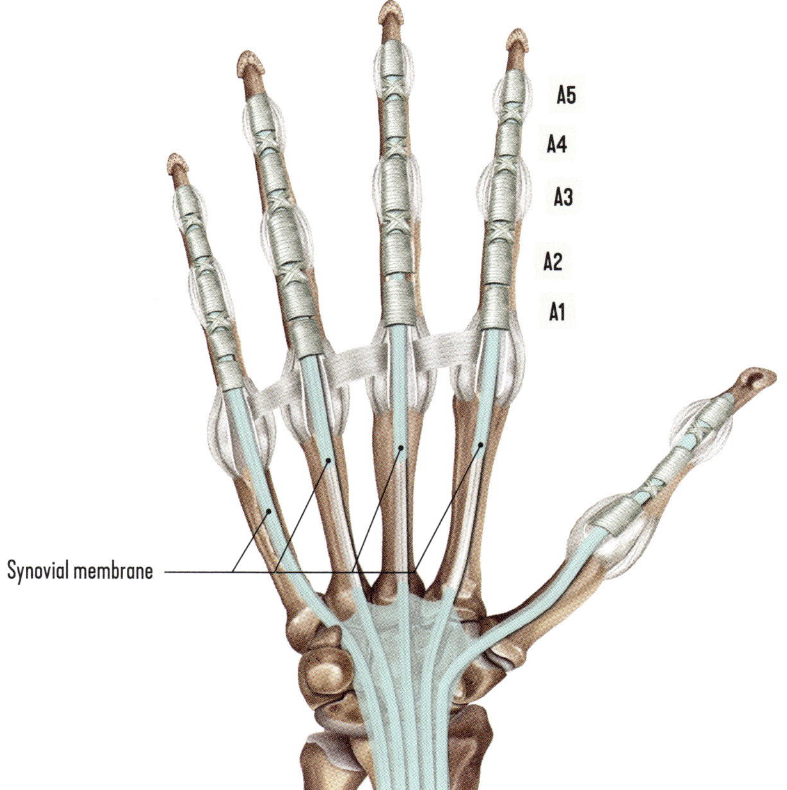

can feel a hard lump over the area in question. This is synovial fluid that has leaked out through a small tear in the synovial membrane and encapsulated itself on the upper side of the tendon sheath. This is called a ganglion cyst.

The cause of tenosynovitis is usually climbing or training too much, either over time or in a single session. The pain can come on gradually, or more acutely after a session where you've worked a lot on hard, finger-heavy boulders or single movements. A lot of crimping is often a contributing factor, as this grip position causes the flexor tendons to push out against the pulleys and pinch the tendon sheath in the middle. A lesser-known cause is climbing a lot on incuts – very positive holds where the edge/lip of the hold presses directly against the tendons and tendon sheath (see page 57). So, both when crimping and when climbing on incuts, the tendon sheath is exposed to compression forces and increased friction between the tendons and the pulleys, and this can cause an inflammatory response in the synovial membrane.

The most important response is to adjust the load and vary grip types. Easier climbing is not necessarily the best option, as many easier climbs – especially indoors – involve climbing on incut jugs and this can further irritate the tendon sheath and pulleys. The solution instead is to climb on smaller or more open holds. By climbing on less steep wall angles you will be able to reduce the load by getting more help from your legs, and by using this approach you can focus on more technically demanding boulders or routes that put less stress on your fingers. If pain permits, you can also climb harder boulders with smaller holds, but be conscious of keeping the sessions shorter and reducing the number of moves per session. I usually recommend to at least halve the session time or session volume, and slowly progress if symptoms don't increase the following day. As with pulley injuries, it is easiest to manage the load by using a fingerboard or a grip tool. You will then be able to use holds and grip positions that don't provoke symptoms, and gradually increase the load. In my experience, the symptoms improve significantly during the warm-up and then return the day after climbing. So, don't be fooled by the fact that it feels better during the session; keep the sessions short and be selective about the choice of hold types and grip positions. If there is no increase in symptoms in the form of increased pain or swelling the day after training, you have found a good balance between training dose and symptom response. The condition will gradually improve, and few need further measures such as a cortisone injection into the tendon sheath.

In recent years, I have recommended patients with tenosynovitis try a simple no-hang protocol once or twice a day, where the goal is to get the synovial fluid to circulate in the tendon sheath and reduce the swelling. The results so far have been good, and it is a simple measure that I recommend alongside managing the load, as described above, and avoiding holds that press directly over the affected area.

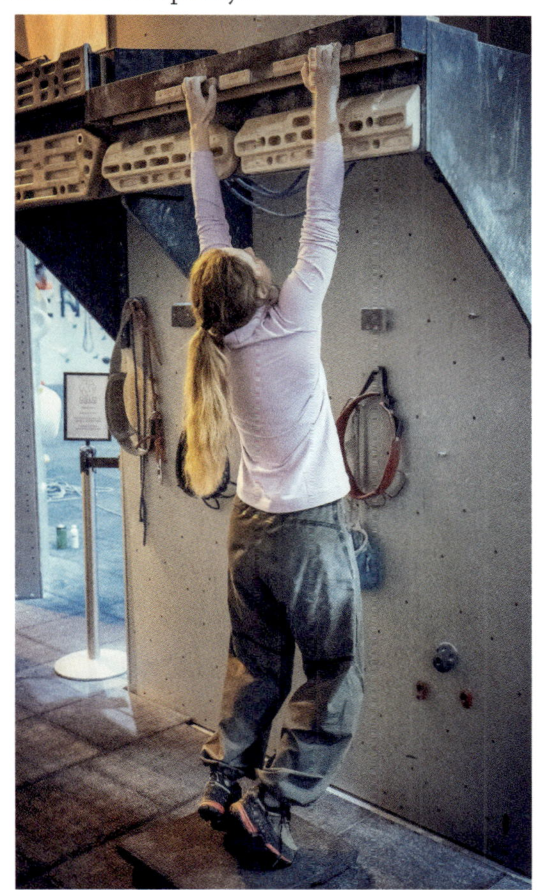

Press your fingers against the grip surface so that you take a few kilos of your body weight. Hold for 10 seconds, rest for 10 seconds, and perform 10 repetitions. Do this once or twice a day.

FINGER JOINTS

'It's here, around the joint in the middle of my finger. It hurts to bend my finger all the way in, and it seems a bit swollen after I've been climbing. I haven't done anything specific lately, but I've been climbing more frequently, and on more fingery routes and boulders.'

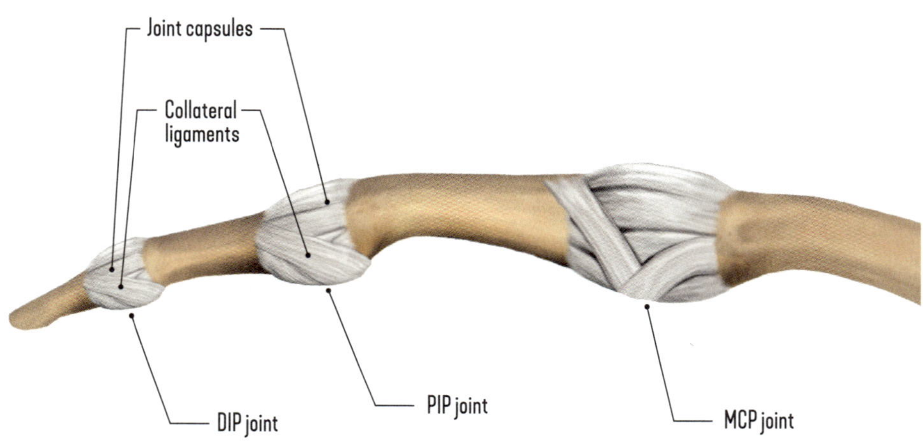

Joint-related issues in the middle and outer finger joints – the PIP (proximal interphalangeal) joints and DIP (distal interphalangeal) joints – are some of the most common reasons why climbers attend my clinic. And it's perhaps not too surprising when we think about it, because when climbing we subject these small joints to high forces on a regular basis. Although we can only actively flex and extend these joints, they can passively rotate and deviate to some extent. The combination of weight and rotational forces that these joints are exposed to can then become too much – both acutely and over time.

MECHANISM OF INJURY

Imagine yourself crimping: the PIP joint is bent to more than 90 degrees, while the DIP joint is *hyperextended*.* Now imagine that the hold you're crimping isn't a horizontal edge but rather an angled grip with an uneven surface. This will subject your finger joints to forces that both rotate and laterally bend them. Thanks to the joint capsules and ligaments surrounding these joints, they will stay in place as long as the forces aren't too great. However, even if the ligaments remain intact, these forces can still cause strains and subsequently reactions in the synovial membrane lining inside a joint capsule. As a result of excessive load over time, or due to an acute incident, inflammation in this synovial membrane – synovitis – leads to increased fluid in the joint space, along with less elastic properties in its capsule. These reactions will make the joint stiffer, and bending and extending the joint will be more difficult; they will also contribute to the experience of pain when loading and moving the joint.

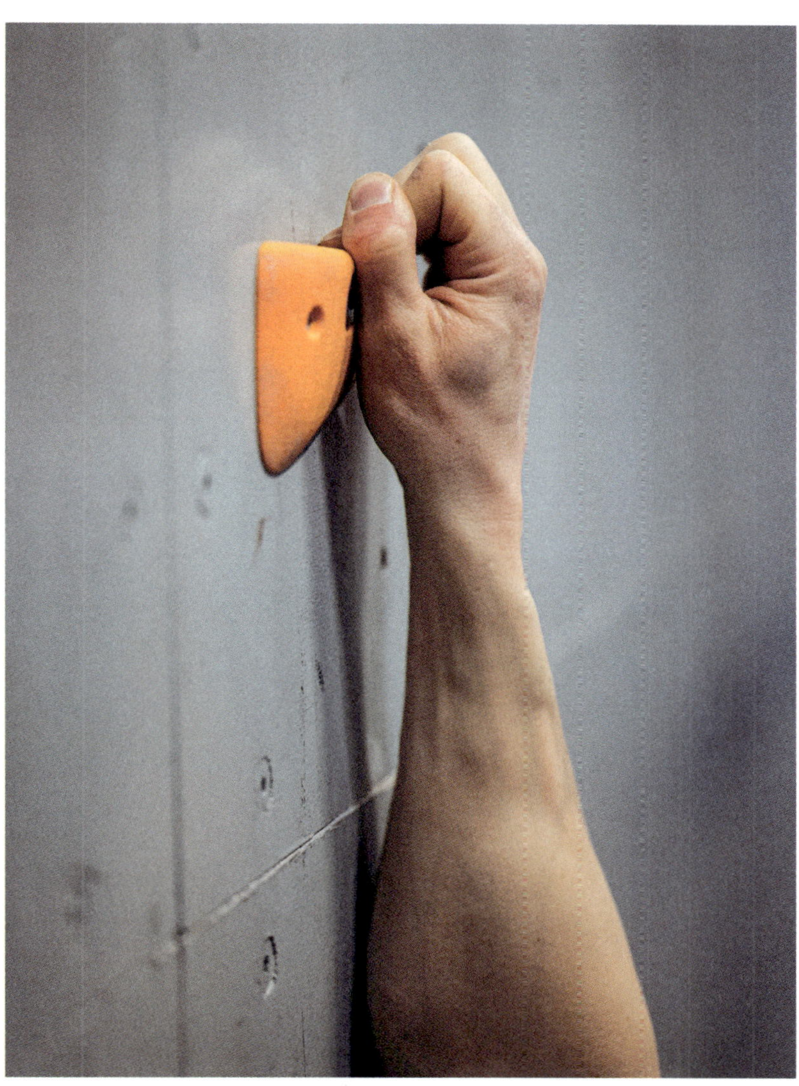

Crimping involves an acute angle in the PIP joints, hyperextended DIP joints and the thumb placed over the index finger.

*Hyperextension means that the joint is overstretched.

MANAGEMENT

It is important to emphasise that if joint pain is related to an acute incident, such as a strain or twist injury from a fall, or from getting a finger caught in a crack or pocket, the stability of the joint should be examined by a healthcare professional. If the collateral ligaments or the joint capsule partially or completely tear because of trauma, the joint must be stabilised with tape or an orthosis (support brace) so that the injury can heal and stability can be restored.

If the joint is not unstable, management will primarily involve load management and awareness of grip positions. By using more open grip positions on less steep wall angles, the load on both the PIP and DIP joints will be significantly reduced compared to steeper climbing with half-crimp and full-crimp grip positions. This allows you to reduce physical intensity while still climbing technically challenging routes and boulders, thereby controlling finger load and instead developing other qualities that can make you a better climber. You can also control the training volume by ending sessions earlier or climbing fewer moves per session, and experience has shown that reducing volume often matters more than reducing intensity.

I often hear climbers say, '*I've been climbing easy routes, but lots of them.*' Paradoxically, this tends to worsen symptoms for two main reasons. The first is that easy routes may not actually be that easy. Even though the grades may be easy, there can still be significant physical stress on your fingers. Imagine an easy route on a steep wall. Your fingers must still bear much of your body weight, and even though the holds are good, it's relatively heavy work. And you will do a lot of it if you climb many routes in one session.

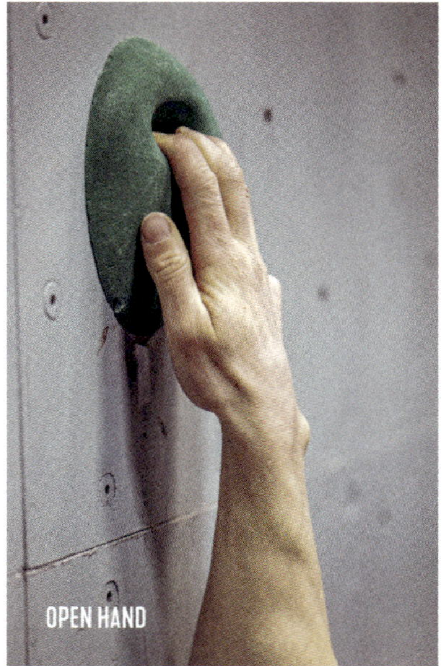

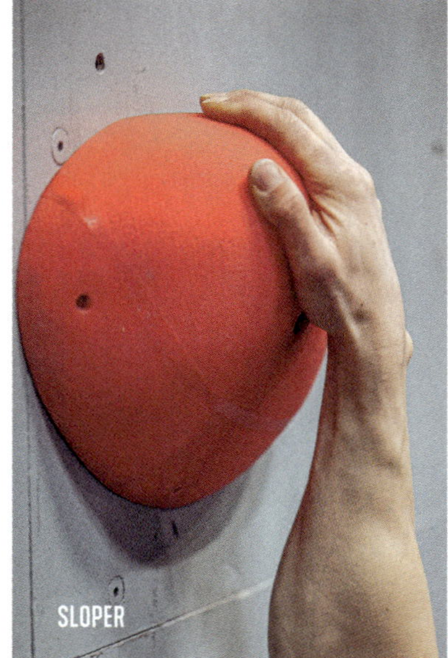

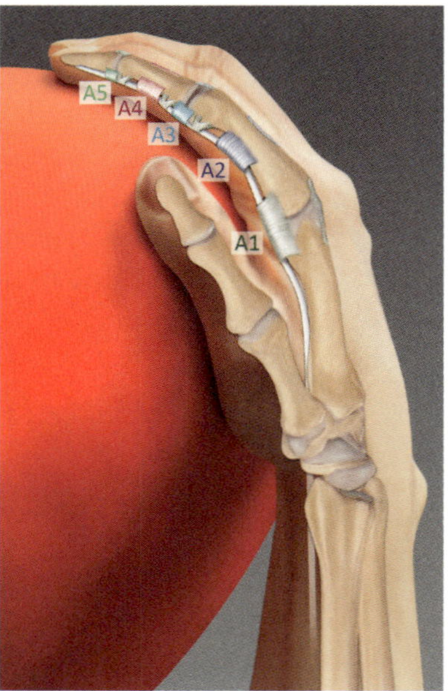

In open grip positions, the DIP and PIP joints are subjected to far less stress than in half-crimp and full-crimp positions. Varying hold selection and grip positions is therefore an important strategy for climbing without provoking symptoms in the finger joints.

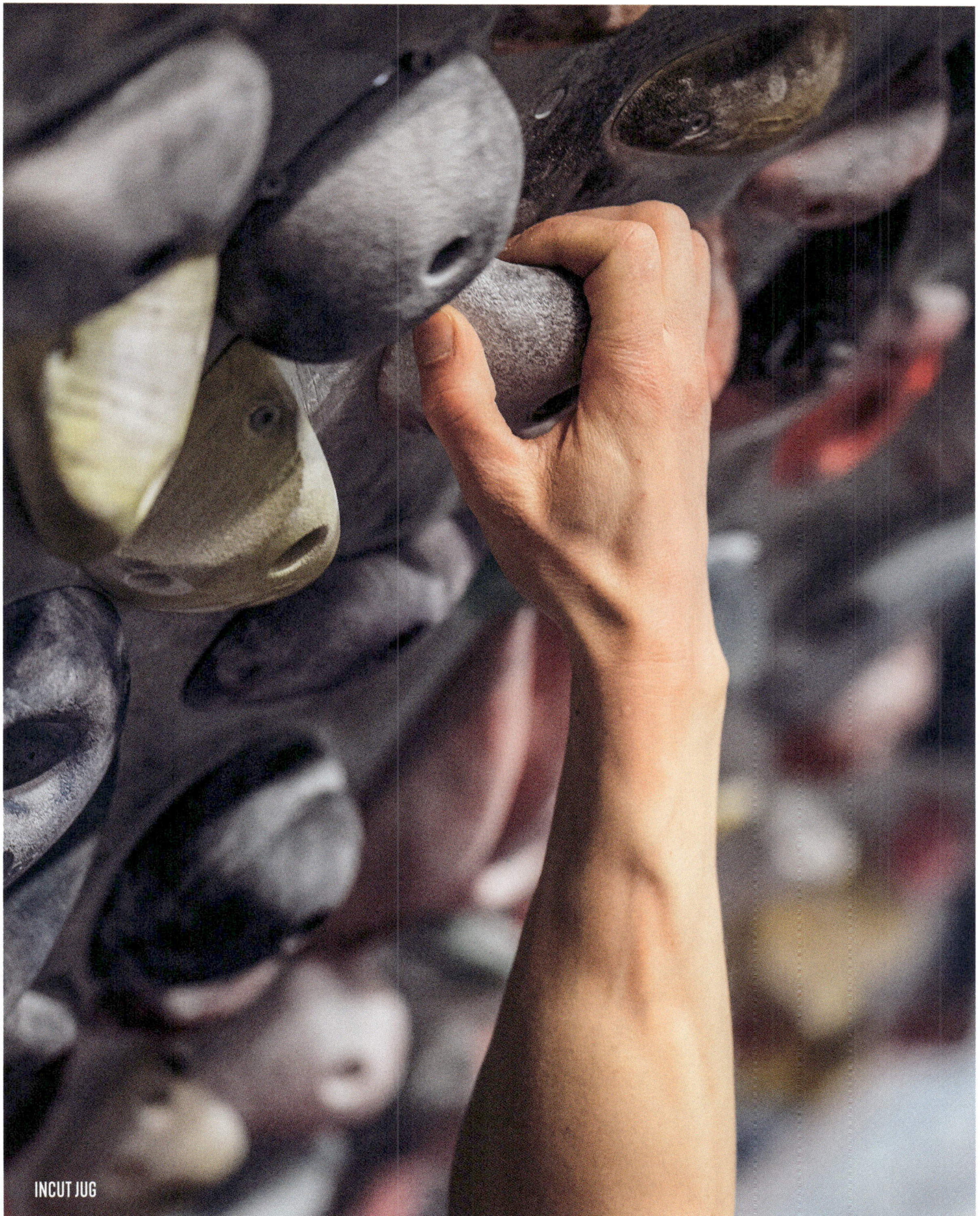

Incut jugs on steeper walls are challenging in several ways. For the PIP joints, this type of hold often leads to the joints being rotated when the weight is moved from the hold. They also provide direct compression against the tendon sheaths in which the flexor tendons lie, thus contributing to the development or maintenance of a condition of inflammation in the tendon sheaths known as tenosynovitis (see pages 52–53).

The second reason is that easier routes or boulders on vertical or steeper walls often have incut holds where the edges of the holds tend to press against the PIP or DIP joints.

Therefore, my recommendation is to initially reduce both volume and intensity when climbing, so that swelling decreases and pain is relieved. Measures such as icing, compression bandages and manual mobilisation of finger joints can be used, with the goal of reducing inflammation, decreasing swelling and increasing mobility. However, at present there are no studies on climbers which demonstrate that these measures have better effects than simply managing load and using the finger in normal day-to-day activities. Nevertheless, these measures have proven effective for synovitis in other joints in the body. If inflammation cannot be reduced with these measures, NSAIDs such as Voltarol and Diclofenac in cream or pill form, as well as cortisone injections directly into the joint, may become relevant interventions.

Deadhangs are a good way to load the fingers under controlled conditions; by keeping volume per session low and hanging in varied grip positions, finger strength can be maintained despite a period of reduced training load. Pain-free training is not a prerequisite, but an increase in swelling afterwards should be avoided; both pain and swelling should return to baseline within 24 hours. This way, you can do several short finger training sessions per week, which could look like this:

- Deadhangs with varied grip positions: 10 seconds on followed by 30 seconds' rest, x5–10 repetitions.

The same principle of avoiding increased swelling will also apply to climbing sessions. As mentioned earlier, focus on gentler wall angles and open grip positions, but once the symptoms are under control, it's natural to resume more finger-intensive training. A key factor will be to keep these sessions short and stop before fatigue sets in.

Looking at the long-term changes that occur in the finger joints of experienced, high-level climbers, it becomes clear that the joints are subjected to high forces over time. These changes involve thicker bones, thicker and stiffer connective tissues, and the formation of osteophytes (bone spurs). However, these changes have not yet been linked to increased pain or reduced activity levels. Joint-related issues function in many ways as a navigational tool for managing load. Handled correctly, you can train around them when they arise, and with awareness of training load and grip positions you can reduce the risk of them occurring in the first place.

DEADHANG SESSION

10 SECONDS' HANG/30 SECONDS' REST, X5–10 REPETITIONS

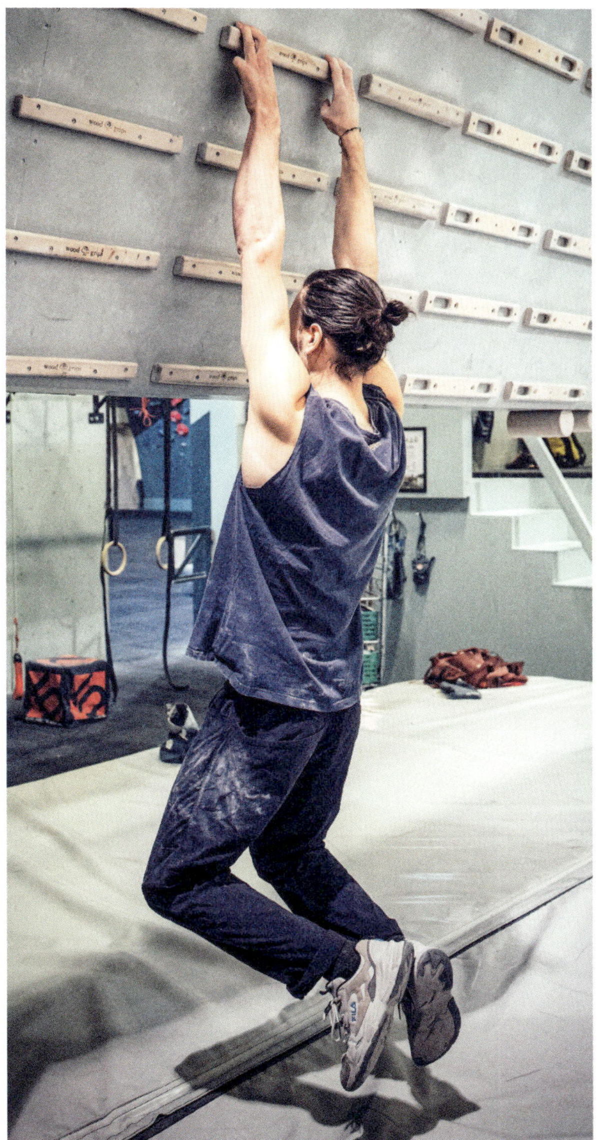

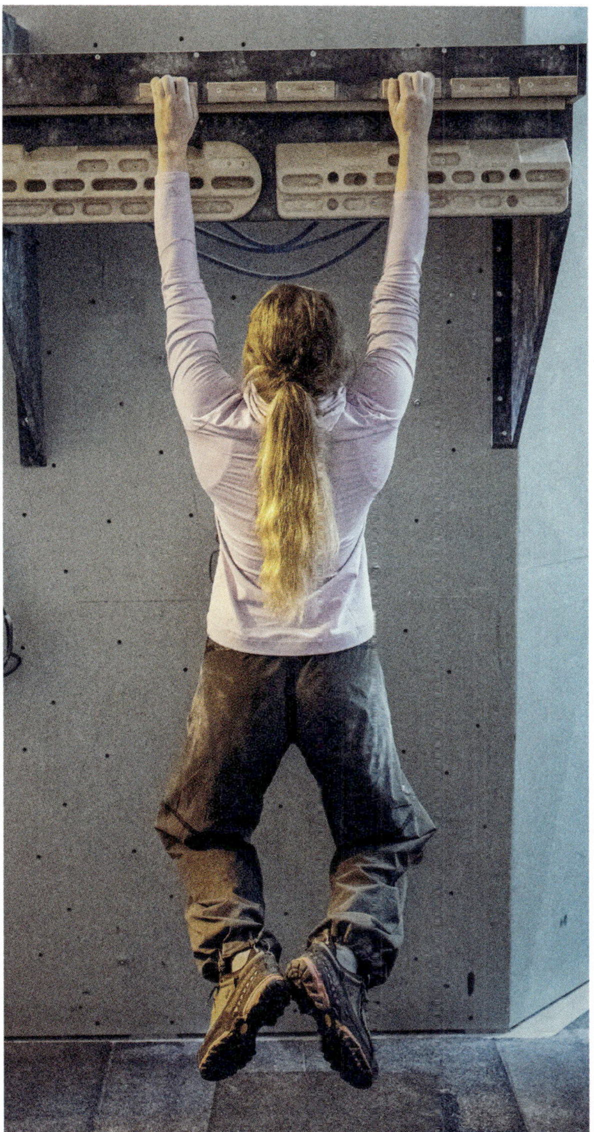

Short hang sessions stimulate the joints while allowing you to build strength in a controlled environment without provoking symptoms; you can vary between different grip positions and choose a weight that suits you. There's nothing wrong with standing with your legs on the floor and doing this as a no-hang protocol if you want to reduce the load even further.

FINGERS: GROWTH PLATE INJURIES

There is one joint-related finger injury that we must handle in a significantly stricter manner: growth plate injuries in younger climbers.

BUT, FIRST AND FOREMOST: WHAT IS A GROWTH PLATE?

In order for our bones to grow in length, they have a growth plate consisting of cartilage tissue at each end. The bones grow in length as the cartilage in the central part of the growth plate expands. Eventually, the new cartilage ossifies and becomes bone tissue, and eventually the growth plate itself also ossifies. The bone is then fully grown but will continue to mature and become thicker and stronger through regular loading.

Until the growth plate is closed and fully ossified, it is the weakest link in the bone-tendon-muscle chain, with the highest risk of injury being during periods of rapid growth in both height and weight. The age at which this period – referred to as *peak height velocity* (PHV) – occurs varies individually, as does when one finishes growing. Most growth plates are fully developed between the ages of 16 and 20, with growth primarily occurring from bottom to top within the body. Therefore, bones in the wrists, hands and fingers are among some of the last to finish growing, which poses challenges for young climbers since their fingers' growth plates are assumed not to be fully ossified until around the ages of 17 to 19.

The majority of adolescents with growth plate injuries are aged 13 to 15, which correlates with when their growth plates begin closing. This closure happens from the inside out, meaning that while the part of the growth plate on the volar side of a finger closes, the part on the dorsal side is still open. This changes how forces distribute through the bone, resulting in injuries on the dorsal aspect where the growth plate has not yet fully ossified. Injuries most commonly occur in the middle (PIP) joint of the middle finger, and are classified as Salter–Harris fractures I–V. The different numbers describe both fracture type and severity, and the most common fracture type in young climbers is Salter–Harris III.

MECHANISM OF INJURY

During crimping, bouldering, campus training and weighted pull-up training on a bar, the growth plates at the PIP joints are exposed to forces that can lead to bone stress reactions, and ultimately fractures, if the load becomes too great. During their early teens, many young climbers increase their training volume and climbing level, while also experiencing rapid growth in both height and mass. It is therefore easy to understand why the risk of injury is high – it is a perfect storm of various factors occurring simultaneously. Awareness of this risk, in the young climbers themselves, and in their coaches and parents, is crucial for adjusting the load young climbers place on their fingers during puberty, and thus reducing their risk of injury.

In some cases, the injury occurs acutely with a noticeable sensation in the finger during climbing. However, in most cases there will be gradually increasing pain and swelling around the PIP joint. Range of motion will be reduced due to swelling and pain, making it painful to fully flex the finger (see photo below). Since these symptoms may develop gradually, and may not always be intense enough during climbing to hinder performance, it is important to recognise them after each session. If you are a young climber and are experiencing such symptoms, it is recommended that you stop climbing and have your finger examined.

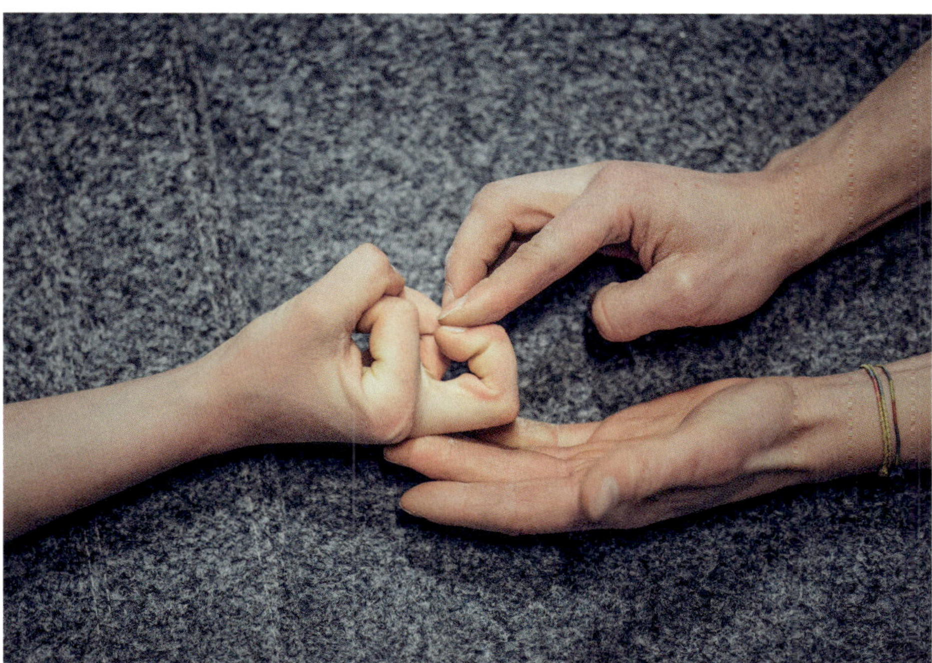

PIP joint provocation test. By pushing the PIP joint into full flexion, it is possible to provoke pain in the event of a growth plate injury. If this is painful, I recommend you take a week off climbing and see if it gets better. If it doesn't improve after a week's rest, I recommend that you have your finger examined more closely to assess the extent of the injury and then make a plan for what to do next.

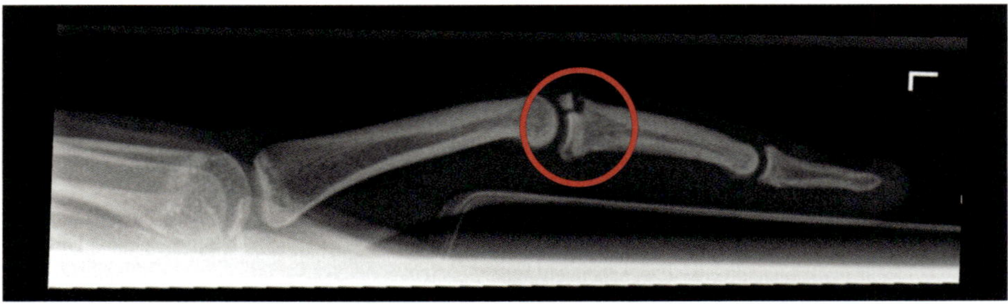

This X-ray shows a Salter–Harris type III injury with a fracture through the growth plate at the PIP joint. By resting the finger for six to eight weeks, the fracture will heal in most cases and the finger will grow back together normally.

MANAGEMENT

When it comes to pain and swelling associated with the PIP joint in younger climbers, there is a high probability that the growth plate is affected. Studies have shown that young climbers experiencing pain and swelling in the PIP joint have a 90 per cent likelihood of having a stress reaction in the growth plate. However, a clinical examination by a healthcare professional familiar with these injuries should be supplemented with an X-ray or MRI scan to assess the severity. If a fracture to the growth plate is observed, the recommended course of action is to rest the finger for six to eight weeks before taking another MRI scan to determine if the fracture has healed.

In rarer cases where there is a displaced fracture – meaning a part of the growth plate has broken loose from the bone – splinting for four to six weeks may be necessary to ensure optimal healing of the fracture. Climbing can be resumed once imaging shows healing, when swelling has subsided, full mobility in the joint has been regained and there is no longer any pain. If, over time, however, the fracture doesn't heal properly, spot-drilling may be considered. This is a technique where small holes are drilled into the bone to allow blood vessels to grow in and contribute to fracture healing. Fortunately, this scenario rarely occurs; if symptoms are taken seriously early on, the finger will fully develop without future problems arising from such injuries. However, if left untreated for too long, the finger will suffer from permanent and irreversible damage, which will ultimately affect finger growth and development and may cause the young person to quit climbing altogether. Finger deformities will also make it difficult to engage in other fine motor activities later in life, emphasising how crucial it is that we take these injuries seriously!

DID YOU KNOW?

Growth plates are also referred to as epiphyseal plates and epiphyseal discs.

Since young climbers are at risk of developing these injuries until the growth plates have ossified, their climbing training during adolescence should be structured to reduce the use of the crimp grip and avoid campus board exercises. Caution should also be exercised when bouldering, particularly avoiding long sessions which focus on finger-intensive bouldering. Fortunately, climbing offers a wide range of possibilities for variation, and engaging in more technically demanding rather than physically demanding climbing in combination with open-handed grip types will serve as good building blocks for developing skills and resilience in the long run. Additionally, there is plenty of physical training for the arms and upper body that does not negatively impact the fingers. Therefore, even with an injury requiring adjustments to finger load, one can emerge from this period as a stronger climber with improved technique.

REMEMBER:

- A growing skeleton is susceptible to growth plate injuries.
- The growth plates in the fingers fully fuse between the ages of 17 and 19.
- Adolescents going through a growth spurt are particularly prone to growth plate injuries, and most of them sustain this injury between the ages of 13 and 15.
- It is usually the PIP joints of the middle fingers that are affected.
- Injuries to growth plates are closely related to the number of climbing hours per week, use of the crimp grip, and specific training methods such as campus boarding and finger-intensive bouldering.
- If there is pain and swelling in the joint, one should take a break from climbing for a week. If symptoms do not improve with this rest period, it is advisable to seek medical attention and have an X-ray or MRI scan of the finger to assess the injury.
- Usually, a rest period of six to eight weeks is recommended before another MRI scan can determine if healing has occurred. If this rehab approach is followed, the prognosis is good, and the climber can expect to return to their previous level within three to four months. However, bear in mind that it may take longer than this, and young climbers and their coaches and parents should be aware of this type of injury throughout adolescence.

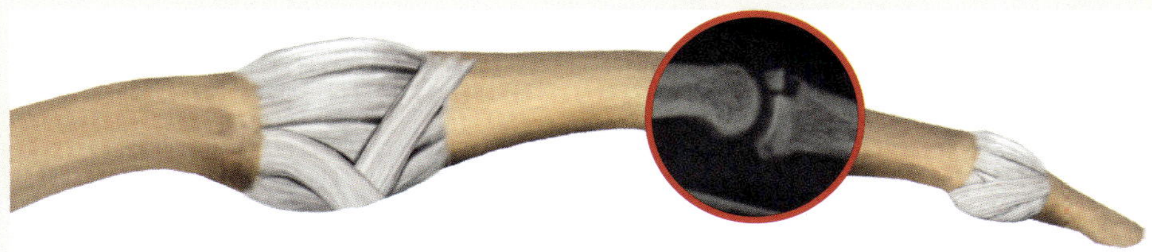

TRAINING, WEIGHT AND NUTRITION IN ADOLESCENCE

During puberty, both body height and body mass increase. Increased body mass leads to increased body weight, thus placing a higher load on the fingers and thereby increasing the injury risk. In girls, this period is estimated to take place between the ages of 11 and 14, and in boys between the ages of 12 and 16. Puberty often coincides with the time when many ambitious young climbers gradually increase their training load, and this combination is not without problems.

Dealing with an increase in body weight during puberty can be very challenging. Many will experience a decline in performance over a period of time, and may feel that their climbing peers are progressing faster than they are. It is particularly unfair for girls, as they don't experience the same muscle growth as boys during puberty and they also tend to gain more fat mass. Therefore, despite putting in the same effort in training, the results may not come as expected, and this obviously affects motivation. Knowledge of how the body develops throughout puberty can help both coaches and athletes adjust their training during certain periods; there are many areas for improvement and development in climbing even if progress in pure muscle strength does not always meet expectations.

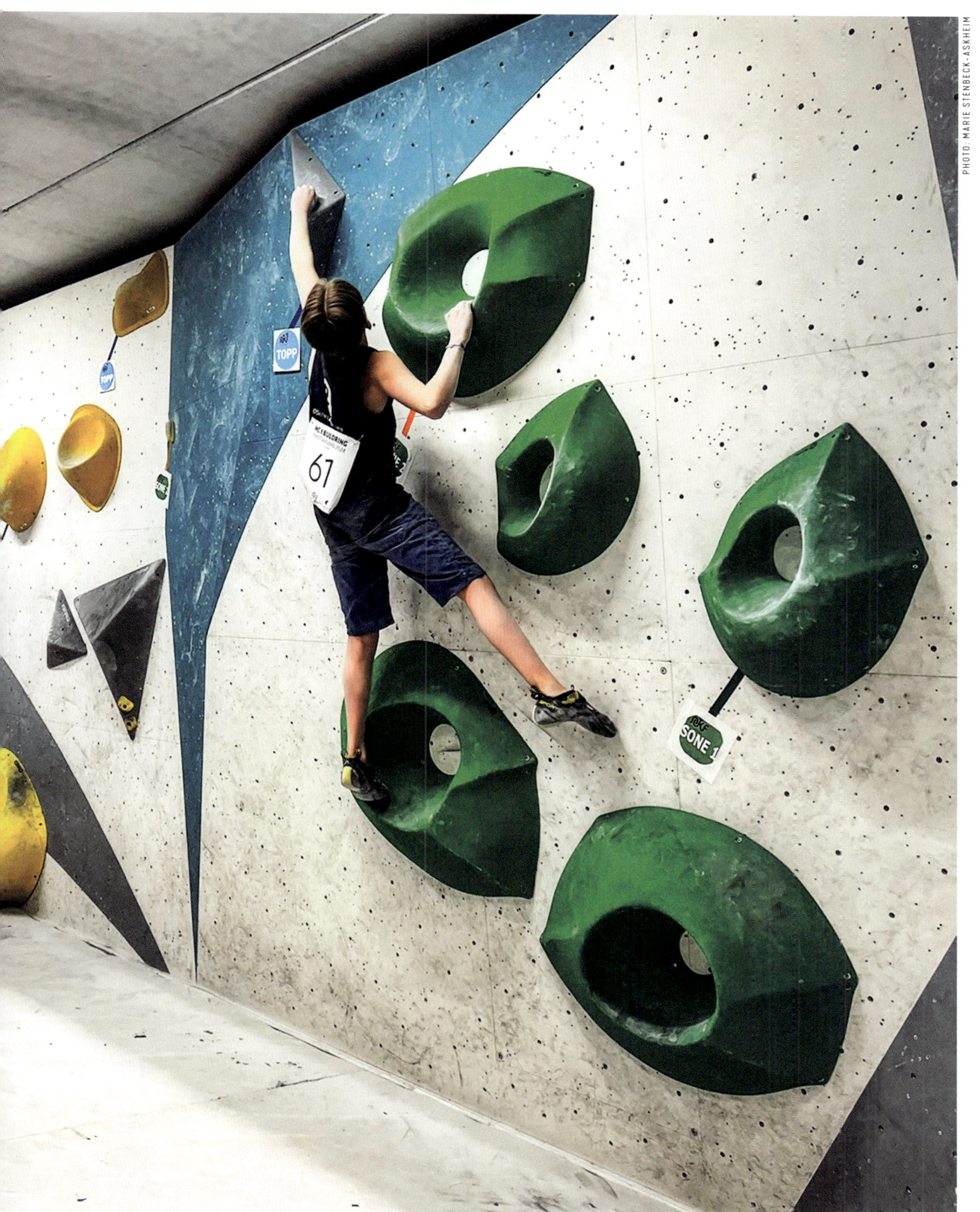

PHOTO: MARIE STENBECK-ASKHEIM

REDs

REDs stands for **Relative Energy Deficiency in Sport**, and occurs when athletes consume less energy than they need. In weight-dependent sports like climbing we can influence the relationship between strength and body weight by becoming stronger or lighter. Reducing weight involves operating at an energy deficit – meaning that we provide the body with less energy than it requires. And, just like going bankrupt where we spend more money than we earn, operating at an energy deficit over time is unsustainable and can lead to serious health consequences.

The interrelationship between low energy availability (with or without disordered eating), menstrual dysfunction (amenorrhea) and low bone mineral density (osteoporosis) is referred to as the *female athlete triad*. The combination of these three components can lead to irreversible health consequences. In some cases, the focus on food and weight can also result in disordered eating or an eating disorder. This is a mental illness that causes both physical and psychological complications for health, and it is potentially fatal. While the female athlete triad only affects women, REDs can occur in both female and male athletes, manifesting as impaired bone health. Additionally, REDs can hinder development in young athletes, weaken the immune system, increase fatigue, increase injury rates, reduce recovery capacity and diminish coordination, strength and concentration.

The use of weight reduction as a performance tool can cause severe physical and psychological injuries that may force individuals to quit climbing. Moreover, it is impossible to train enough – or well enough – over time if constantly operating at an energy deficit. Eventually, fitness levels will decline significantly, and it's often difficult to regain previous levels of performance through training alone. Many people lack the motivation required for this process and therefore they end up quitting climbing instead. It's extremely important to establish a healthy training environment, where young climbers are allowed to develop at their own pace and where nutrition and puberty are natural topics of discussion. This way we can reduce the risk of early performance-oriented goals, where weight reduction is used as a means along the way.

However, it is important to emphasise that REDs does not necessarily have to exist alongside an eating disorder or arise as a result of desired weight loss. It can also be related to the energy available for exercise. If you haven't eaten enough when you use more energy, your body won't be able to maintain all its functions.

So, even if you're not intentionally trying to lose weight or you see a weight reduction on the scales, it's possible that you still aren't getting enough energy. This is important to be aware of for younger athletes, who have high energy demands as they grow and often have busy schedules and may forget to eat along the way.

The Norwegian Olympic and Paralympic Committee and Confederation of Sports has a priority programme called *Healthy Sports*. It has listed characteristics that one can look out for which indicate a risk of developing REDs:

- disordered eating behaviour
- strong focus on perfectionism regarding food and exercise
- recurring infections and illnesses
- frequent injuries
- stress reactions/stress fractures in the skeleton
- menstrual disorders
- decreased libido

If you can identify with several of these points, it is important to ask yourself the following questions:

1. Am I exercising too much?
2. Am I eating enough/often enough?
3. Am I allowing enough time for rest and recovery?

This section started with a discussion of stress reactions in the growth plates of the finger joints, and ended by discussing growth, weight and nutrition. Growth plate injuries can occur due to a growing body being combined with increased training load alone, but it's important that we have an awareness of growth, weight and nutritional issues in young climbers. Almost all injuries are a result of multiple factors, and the most important thing we should ensure is that young climbers take care of their health and lay a solid foundation for climbing as a lifelong activity.

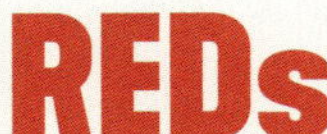

REDs

Relative Energy Deficiency in Sport

WHAT IS IT?

A condition of energy deficiency causing adverse effects on all bodily systems. It affects both male and female athletes who do not fuel adequately, whether intentionally or not.

RECOGNITION & NEXT STEPS

- Perfectionist tendencies
- Disordered/restricted eating
- Frequent injuries/niggles
- Illness
- Menstrual dysfunction
- Loss of sex drive

ARE YOU ...

- Overtraining?
- Fuelling adequately?
- Taking regular rest days?

SEEK MEDICAL HELP

- GP can rule out other conditions
- GP can refer to specialist services

WHY DOES IT MATTER?

1. Impaired growth and development
2. Impact on health and well-being
3. Adverse effect on performance

FOR FEMALE ATHLETES:

- Regular menstrual cycle is a barometer of hormone health.
- Not starting periods by age 16, or not having periods for >6 months requires medical investigation.
- Oral contraceptive pill (OCP) can mask problems without providing bone protection or addressing underlying cause.
- Using OCP for contraception needs to be an informed decision by the athlete.

BE AWARE THAT ...

20%

Prevalence of disordered eating is 20% higher among athletes compared to non-athletes.

Dudgeon, Emily, 'Relative energy deficiency in sport (RED-S): recognition and next steps', 2019, BMJ blog (22 April 2019), https://blogs.bmj.com/bjsm/2019/04/22/relative-energy-deficiency-in-sport-red-s-recognition-and-next-steps Reprinted with permission.

8 TRAINING RECOMMENDATIONS FOR YOUNG CLIMBERS:

1. Make training varied and enjoyable.
2. Focus on many moves rather than hard moves.
3. Spend most of the training time learning technical fundamentals and developing good movement patterns on the wall.
4. Train strength for the arms and upper body but pay careful attention to the training methods used for specific finger strength training. Focus on technical execution, simple training methods, low training volume and gradual progression.
5. Use basic strength and conditioning training for overall body strength, as well as balance, coordination and endurance training.
6. Eat healthy food, eat enough and eat regularly.
7. Pay attention to any symptoms in the fingers throughout puberty, but especially during periods of rapid increase in height and body mass.
8. BE PATIENT!

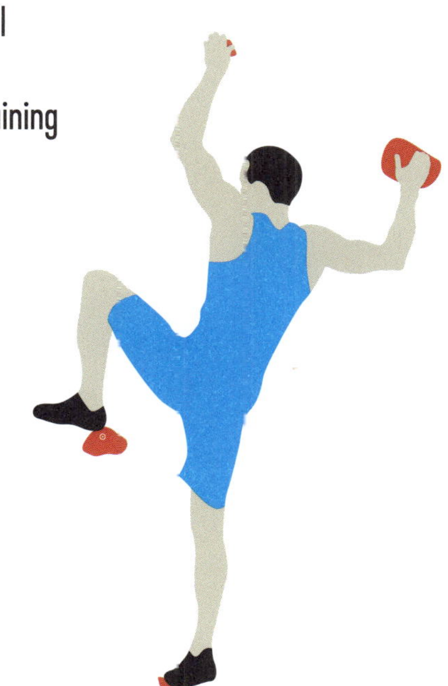

FLEXOR MUSCLES AND LUMBRICALS

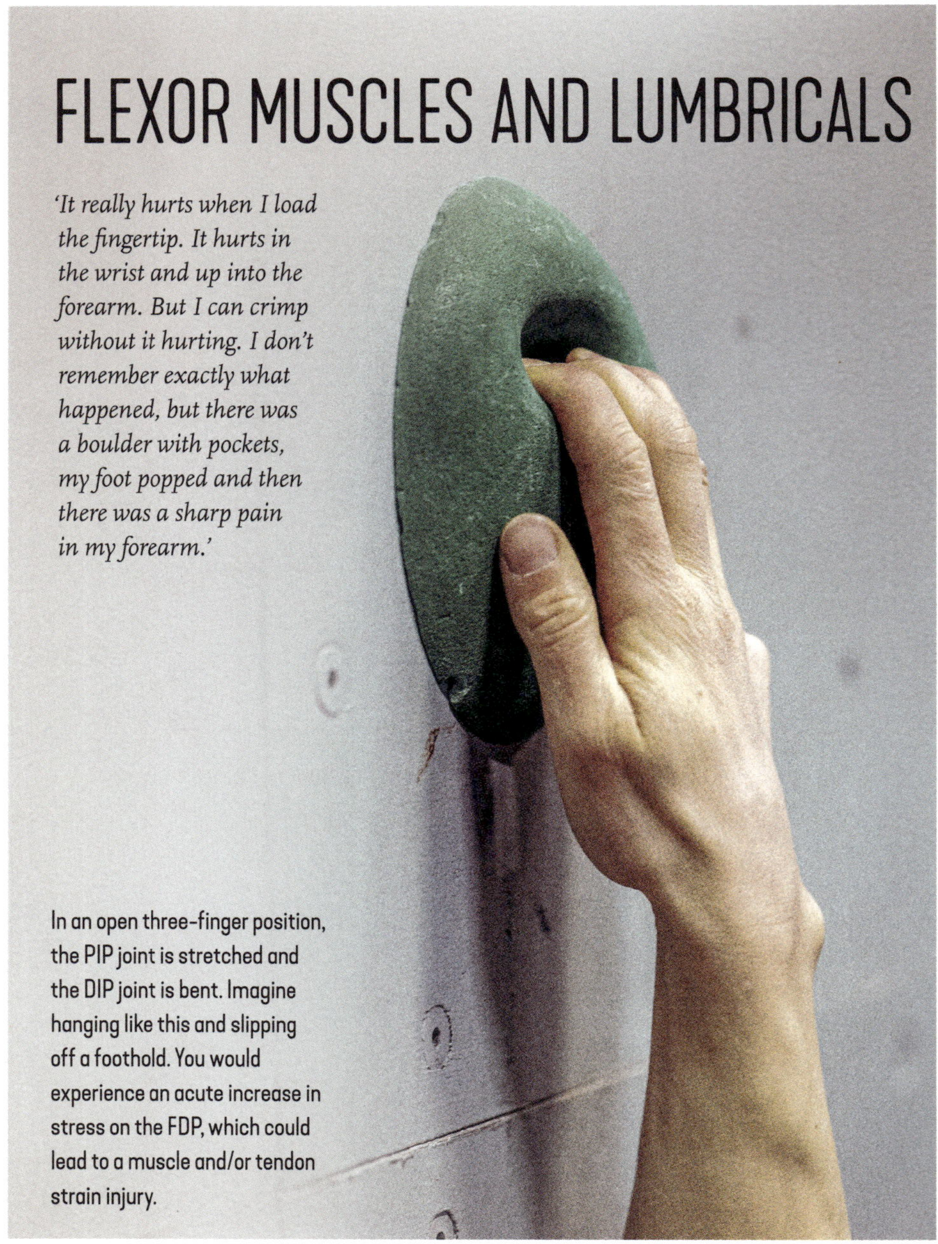

'It really hurts when I load the fingertip. It hurts in the wrist and up into the forearm. But I can crimp without it hurting. I don't remember exactly what happened, but there was a boulder with pockets, my foot popped and then there was a sharp pain in my forearm.'

In an open three-finger position, the PIP joint is stretched and the DIP joint is bent. Imagine hanging like this and slipping off a foothold. You would experience an acute increase in stress on the FDP, which could lead to a muscle and/or tendon strain injury.

We have two sets of muscles that flex the fingers, the flexor digitorum superficialis (FDS) and the flexor digitorum profundus (FDP). The former bends the middle (PIP) finger joint, and the latter bends the outermost (DIP) finger joint. In an open grip position (see photo above), the middle joint is extended while we bend at the outermost joint; this means that the FDP must bear most of the load in this grip position.

MECHANISM OF INJURY AND DIAGNOSIS

With a sudden increase in load – such as from a foot popping, your pinky finger slipping off while in a four-finger half crimp, or latching a hold in an open two- or three-finger position – you can sustain a strain injury to either the muscle, the tendon, or both. It is usually the ring finger that is affected, since for most people it is shorter than their index and middle fingers; while the ring finger remains straight at its PIP joint, the other two fingers still maintain some degree of flexion at their PIP joints. With a muscle strain injury, pain will be localised to the wrist and forearm, as this is where the muscle mass is located. A tendon strain injury can be a partial or a complete rupture; a total rupture of the FDP will leave you unable to flex the DIP joint. Fortunately, tendon injuries are far less common compared with muscle injuries which occur relatively frequently. I say fortunately, because tendon ruptures require a longer healing time, and surgery in severe cases, whereas muscle injuries heal relatively quickly. A clinical examination, supplemented by ultrasound examination if necessary, will provide insight regarding the severity of the injury, and this is important for determining the best course of action.

Muscle injuries are graded based on the degree of tissue damage, referred to as a rupture or tear. There is currently no literature specifically grading strain injuries in the FDP, but clinical experience suggests that most injuries are minor muscle ruptures. This corresponds to grade 1 in the general classification of muscle injuries.

CLASSIFICATION OF MUSCLE INJURIES

There are various grading tables for muscle injuries, but Pollock and colleagues' table from 2014 (below) is the most recent and is also well documented. Each of the numerical gradings can be further divided into a, b or c, depending on where the injury occurs within the muscle-tendon unit, and this will have implications for rehabilitation time: a muscle injury involving parts of the tendon (type c) will take longer to heal than injuries limited to the muscle belly and muscle-tendon (myotendinous) junction (MTJ) (types a and b).

British Athletics muscle injury classification	Grade 1 (small tear)	Increasing severity of symptom, signs and radiological disturbance
	Grade 2 (moderate tear)	
	Grade 3 (extensive tear)	
	Grade 4 (complete tear)	

MANAGEMENT

The positive thing about these injuries is that you can keep training and climbing, as long as you hang and climb with four fingers. When you place the pinky finger on a hold, you must bend the PIP joints in the other three fingers. By doing this, you engage the FDS, in addition to protecting the FDP from the direct strain it receives in the open three-finger grip position. This allows you to start loading the injured muscle early on, which is important for ensuring optimal healing and maintaining your existing physical capacity. The most controllable way to start the rehabilitation is by using a fingerboard or a grip tool, using a four-finger half-crimp position. This gives you control over the grip position and the number of kilos added, allowing you to adjust the load based on your symptom response. It is also important to use an open grip position to specifically target the FDP, and by using the same tools, you can easily reduce the weight from a four-finger half crimp and use three, two or one fingers in an open grip position. The progression ladder is similar to that after pulley injuries (see pages 49–51), but this time in open grip positions.

As with all muscle injuries, there is a risk of re-injury if you progress too fast; therefore, it's important to have control over grip position, load and movement tempo during rehabilitation. Based on experience, full recovery can be expected within six to eight weeks if recurring strains are avoided during this period.

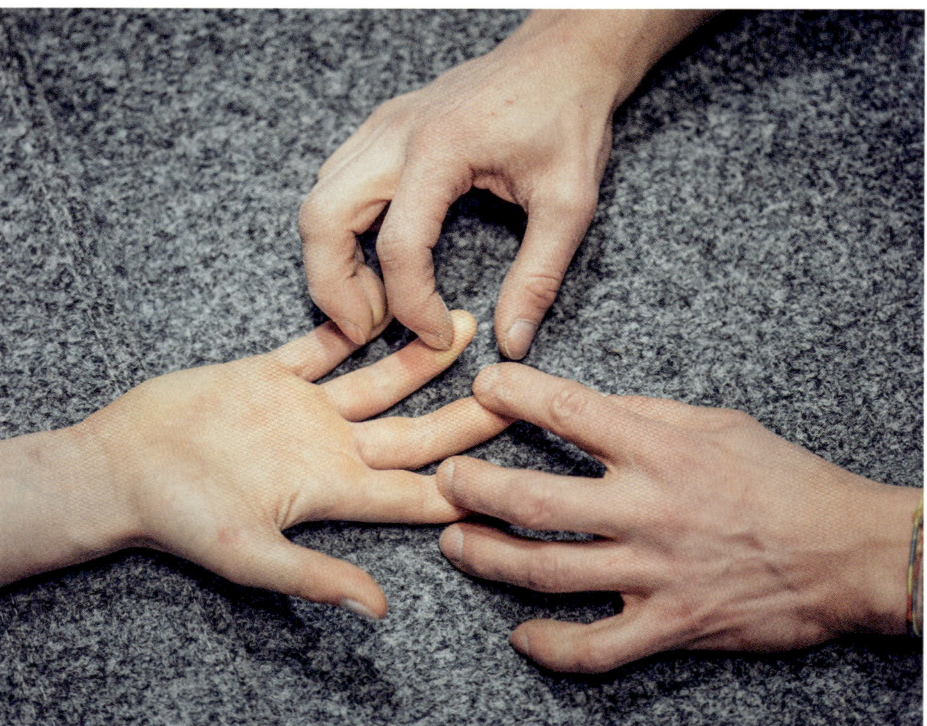

This photo shows a test of the deep flexor muscle (FDP) of the ring finger. With the other fingers straight, the fingertip is pressed against resistance while the PIP joint is stretched. Pain in the forearm and wrist indicates a strain to the FDP.

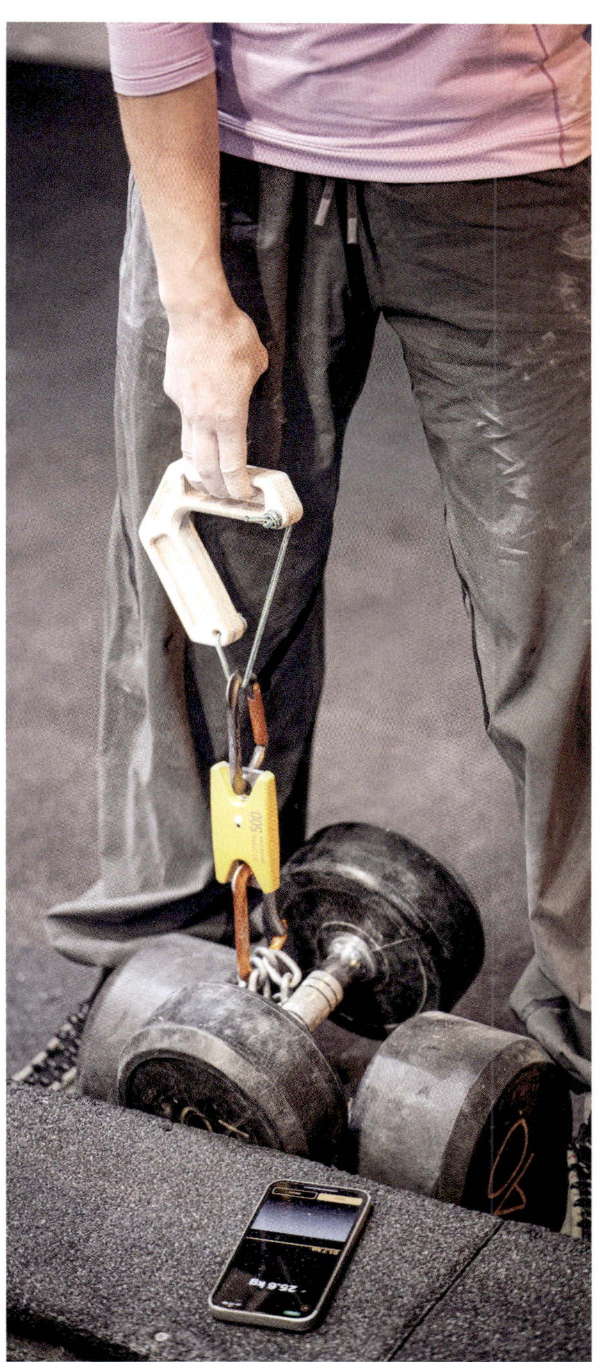

After an injury, it's important to load with an open grip to give your muscles a specific stretch. By using a grip tool and a load cell, you can control the load and the speed of the movement, and pull as hard as you feel comfortable.

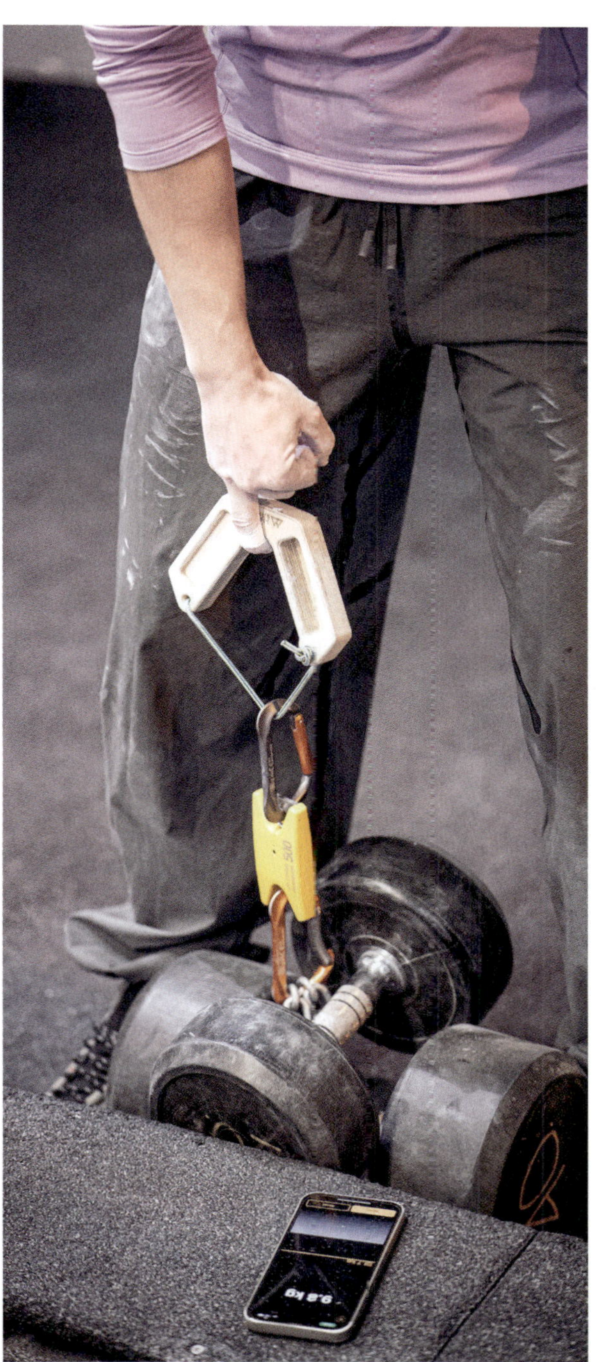

This grip position can be used to train both the FDP and the lumbricals (see next page).

LUMBRICAL SHIFT SYNDROME

The lumbrical muscles are located in the palm of the hand, and are attached to the flexor tendons. When we climb on pockets, the neighbouring fingers to the ones being used will automatically flex to generate more force. This results in a 'shift', where one flexor tendon shortens while the neighbouring tendon lengthens, causing the lumbrical muscle that is attached to both tendons to stretch. The majority of injuries are classified as grade 1 or 2 muscle injuries and are initially diagnosed through clinical examination. In cases where one suspects more extensive muscle/tendon damage, an ultrasound examination can be performed to supplement the diagnosis. This injury can occur independently, but it is often seen in conjunction with injuries to the flexor muscles, as described on the previous pages. The pain is localised in the palm, but as with injuries to the flexor muscles, it may be possible to climb without symptoms using four fingers in a half-crimp or full-crimp position.

Rehabilitation follows the same progression as for injuries to the flexor muscles, but it may be appropriate to tape the fingers to reduce the risk of re-injury. During acute phases, buddy taping is recommended, while more extensive injuries might require a taping technique which reduces how much the neighbouring fingers can bend.

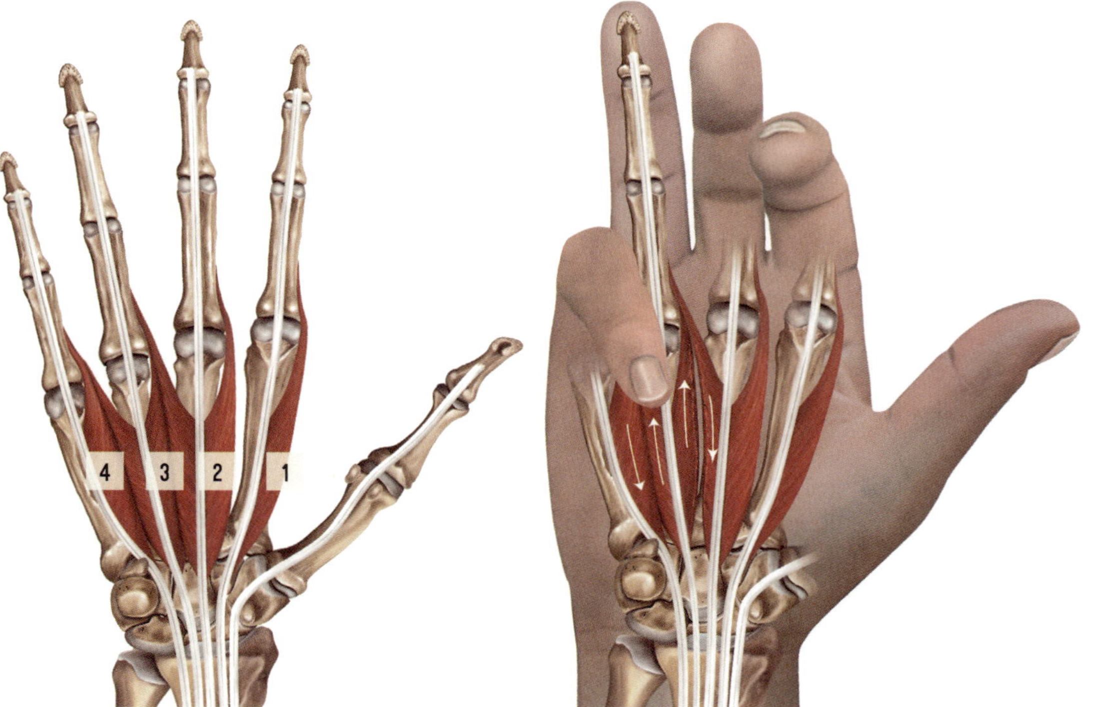

The 3rd and 4th lumbricals are most susceptible to injury because they are attached to two flexor tendons. If the ring finger tendon is stretched at the same time as the pinky finger tendon is shortened, the 4th lumbrical is stretched in two directions and can be damaged if the forces are great enough.

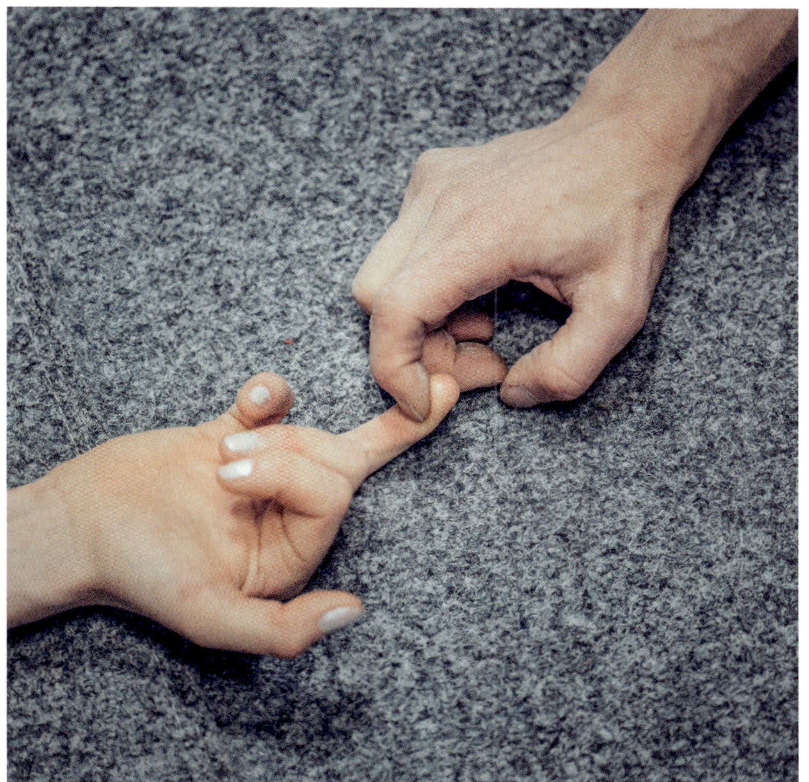

STRESS TEST FOR THE LUMBRICALS. Press the tip of the finger against resistance with the PIP joint extended and the other fingers flexed towards the palm. Pain in the palm over the relevant lumbrical muscles indicates a strain injury.

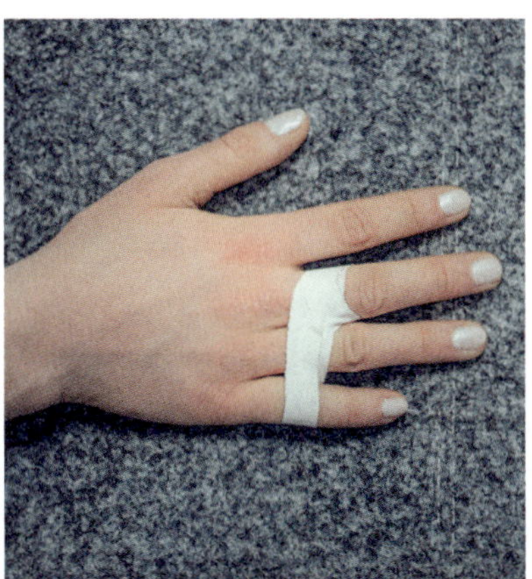

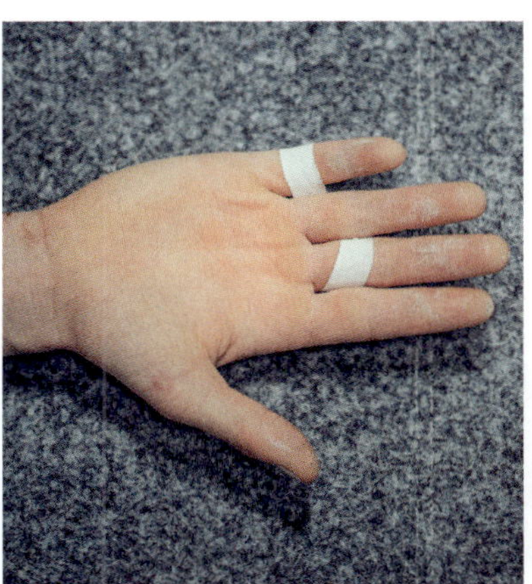

This method of taping allows more freedom of movement, but also limits the amount of flexion and extension of the three fingers in relation to each other. When recovering from a major lumbrical injury, this taping can be used to reduce the risk of recurrence when climbing.

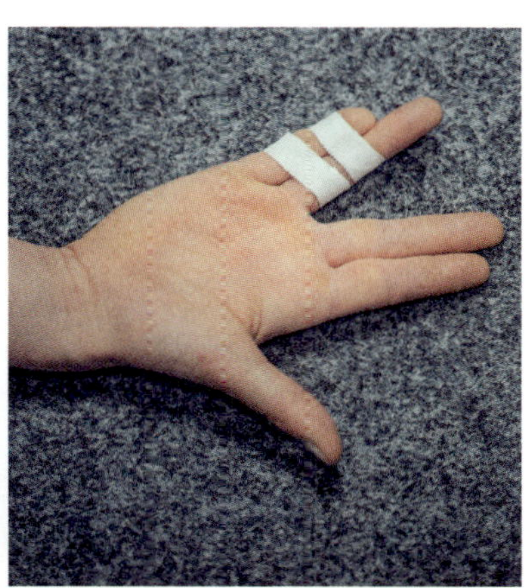

Buddy taping prevents the pinky finger from bending inwards, thus preventing a lumbrical shift between the ring and pinky fingers.

DUPUYTREN'S CONTRACTURE

This is not actually an injury, but a condition that can be influenced and caused by several factors – such as genetics, diabetes and manual labour – and is traditionally observed in men aged between 40 and 60. However, climbers also experience it at a younger age, probably due to the stress we put on the connective tissue in the palms of our hands.

This connective tissue – called the palmar aponeurosis – can then contract so that it feels like a hard lump in the palm of the hand, usually in relation to the ring or little fingers. For most people, this is the only symptom, but in more severe cases, this contracture will cause the ring finger to remain flexed at its base (MCP) joint, and surgery may be considered if there's a fixed and significant contracture of the finger. It seems that there is little we can do to prevent or treat this condition beyond maintaining a healthy lifestyle and trying to maintain mobility with stretching exercises if symptoms do occur. However, it is a harmless condition that should not require taking a break from climbing unless surgery becomes necessary.

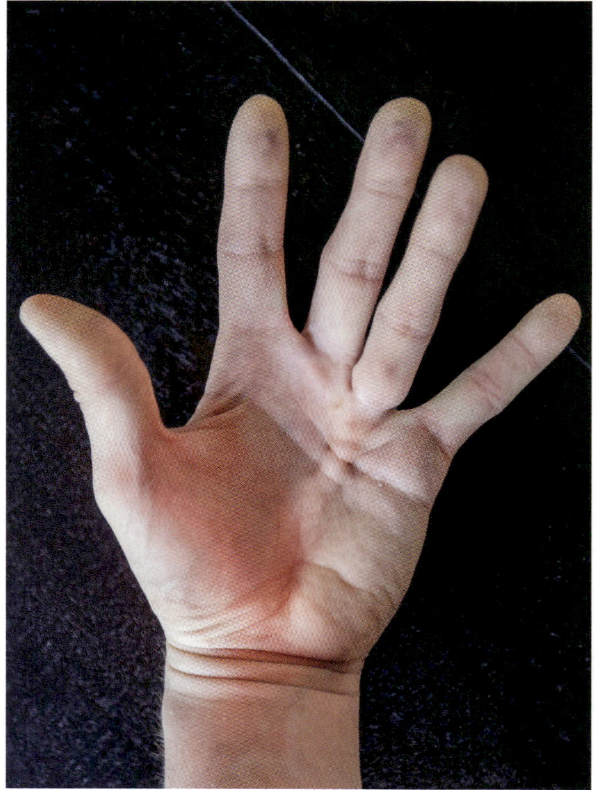

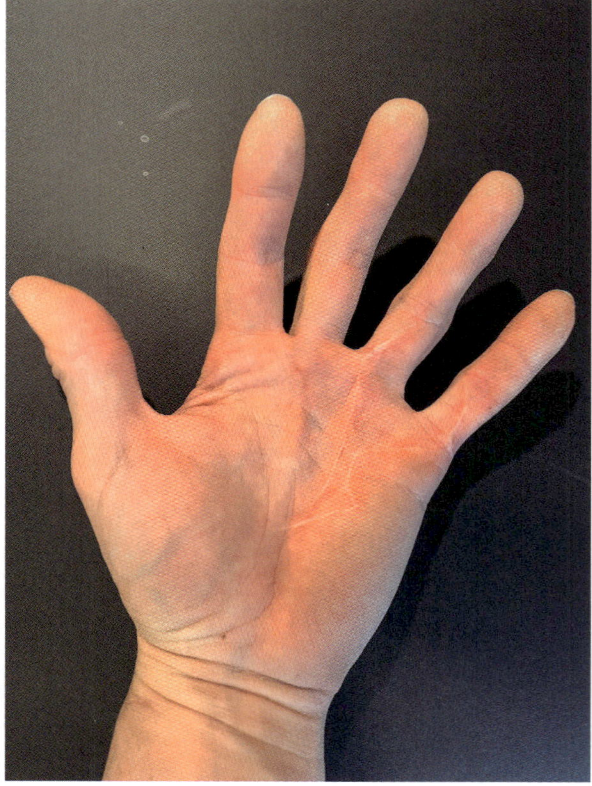

DUPUYTREN'S CONTRACTURE. In this case, the misalignment in the ring finger became significant enough that surgery was necessary.

HANDS AND WRISTS

The wrist is formed by the forearm bones – radius and ulna – and the carpal bones of the hand. The ulnar side of the wrist refers to the pinky finger side, while the radial side refers to the thumb side.

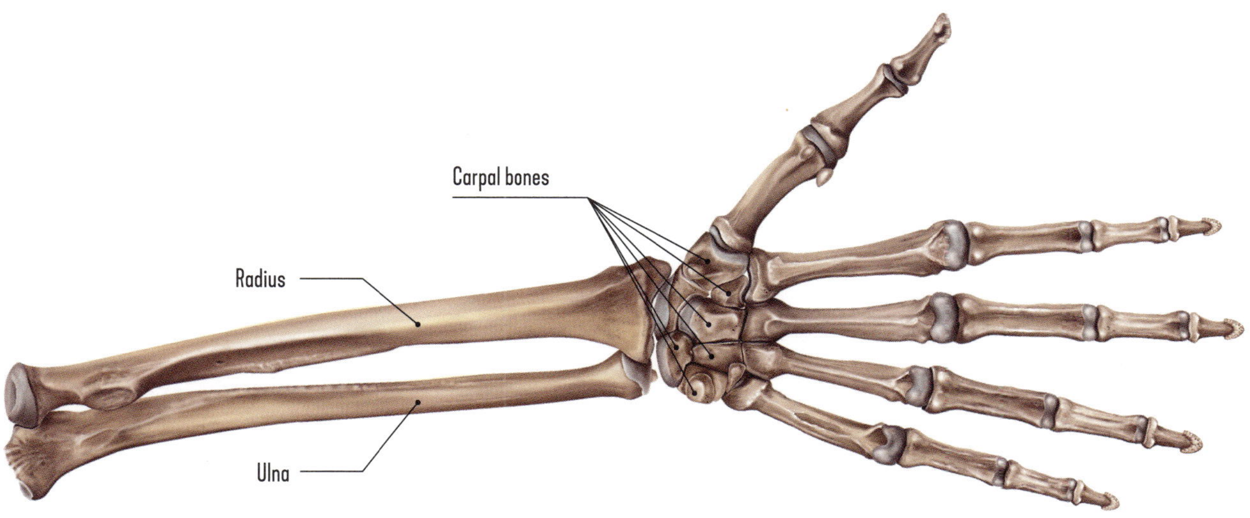

Climbing-related problems in the wrist range from acute and severe injuries, to load-related issues which will only require a change in loading pattern. To distinguish between these, we must first be aware of where in the wrist it hurts and how the problem has arisen.

REPETITIVE STRAIN INJURIES IN THE WRIST

Symptoms that arise gradually are usually related to irritation or inflammation (synovitis) in the wrist, or bone marrow oedema in the forearm and/or carpal bones. Bone marrow oedema can be compared to a bruise on a bone, caused by compression of the joint surfaces. Synovitis is the inflammation of the synovial membrane due to high stress within the joints (see pages 52–53).

Pain is most often located on the ulnar side of the wrist, which is not surprising considering how we flex our wrists towards the ulnar side when we grip. In some cases, such as 'wrapping' a volume (see overleaf) or twisting into an undercut, this flexion combines with a rotation of the wrist, stressing the joint to a high degree. The same stress occurs during a mantelshelf, when we place much of our body weight on to our palms and push up.

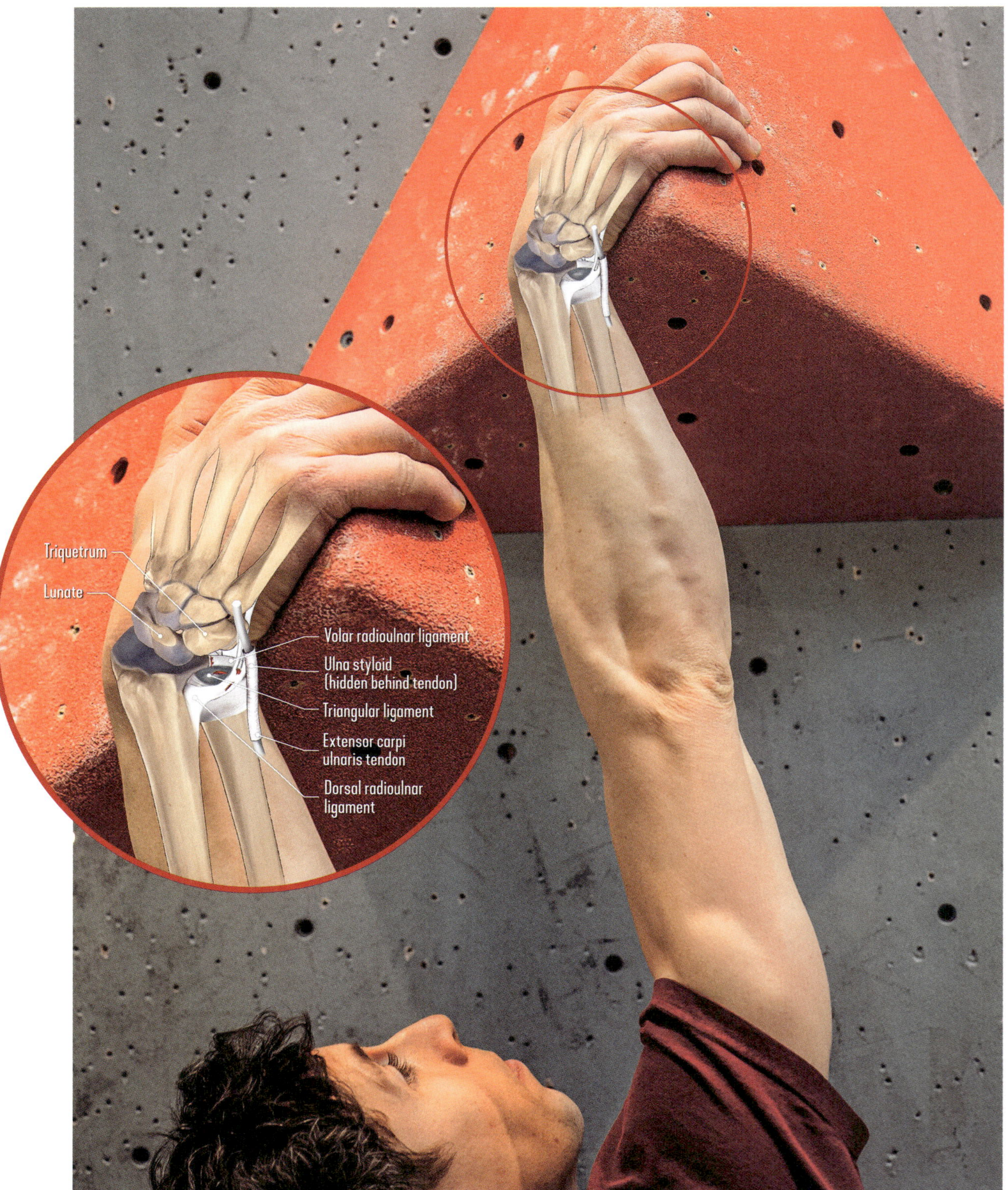

Triangular volumes and large holds invite you to 'wrap' your hands around the edge. As the pictures show, this exposes the wrist to both rotation and lateral flexion, while at the same time providing a firm grip.

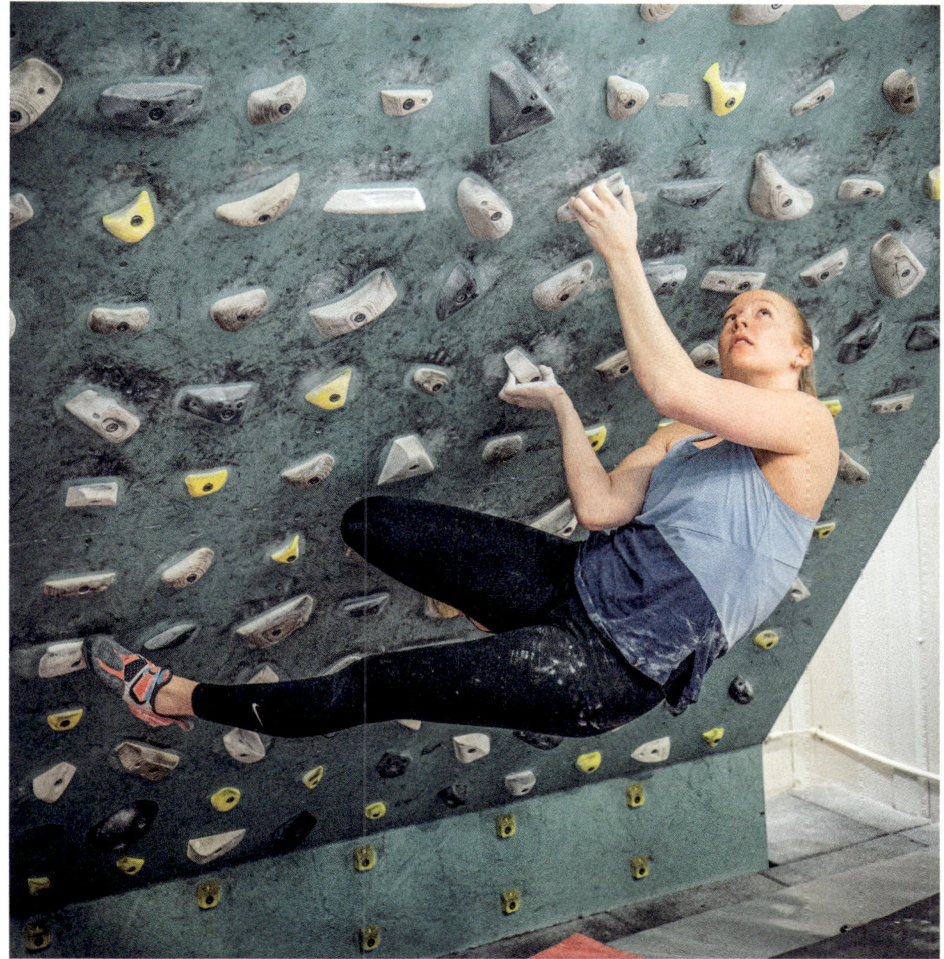

Twisting into an undercut and then moving out of that position requires a combination of wrist extension and lateral flexion towards the pinky finger side.

Bone marrow oedema can be detected by MRI, while synovitis presents as increased fluid on ultrasound images of the wrist. However, imaging diagnostics are not necessary if these problems were not triggered by an acute trauma as it's unlikely that the course of rehabilitation will change because of any potential findings on imaging.

The rehabilitation approach involves adjusting loading patterns and continuing training without a worsening of symptoms afterwards. Adjusting loading patterns means being selective about grip positions and movements. If mantels cause pain, it's okay to avoid boulders or routes with difficult mantels for now. If a project involves using a sidepull or an undercut, and wrist pain is felt after a few attempts, instead work on other parts of the project or take a short break from it. Learning to train on a spray wall allows you to easily vary hold/grip type, wall angle and move length, enabling quality training without worsening symptoms. By using smaller holds, doing shorter moves, improving foot placements and using less steep wall angles, you have many options to help you to adapt the load on your wrists while still having great climbing sessions.

ACUTE WRIST INJURIES

Acute injuries, however, resulting from a fall on a hand or a sudden incident during a move, should be further investigated. There are several stabilising structures, especially on the ulnar side of the wrist, that can be damaged, leading to both structural instability in the wrist and recurrent synovitis. The most well known of these structures is the *triangular fibrocartilage complex* (TFCC), which is attached to the ulna and the carpal bones. This complex binds together the bones of the forearm and stabilises the wrist on its ulnar side. The most common mechanism of injury is falling on to an outstretched arm while using the hand for support. More relevant to us climbers is the stress this complex undergoes when we angle our wrist towards the pinky side of the wrist and rotate our forearm – again, think how the wrist is angled in an undercut position. If you experience an acute incident in such a gripping position, followed by pain and a feeling of instability and/or clicking on the ulnar side of your wrist, I recommend that you have it further evaluated. This can be done through a clinical examination, and be supplemented with an MRI scan.

Some types of TFCC injuries require surgical intervention, but, generally speaking, both acute and load-related TFCC injuries are treated with load management and training. The preferred approach is to avoid positions that provoke symptoms – which usually involve flexing towards the pinky side with or without rotation – while simultaneously working on regaining strength and mobility. However, you must expect symptoms to persist throughout this process, which can last for several months, and for improvement to be gradual and slow. To help stabilise the wrist during rehabilitation, you can use tape or orthoses to increase stability. In cases of recurrent synovitis, cortisone injections may be considered as an option to reduce inflammation and facilitate further rehabilitation.

Being aware that certain grip positions make the wrist more exposed to overuse and injury is the most important preventive measure you can take. You can then consider whether it is necessary to make that famous last attempt, or you can try adjusting your body position so that the wrist is in a less vulnerable position. Through systematic strength training, the wrist will be able to tolerate higher forces, and you will be able to maintain a more favourable joint position in the wrist while climbing. Specifically strengthening the wrist appears central to a reduction in the risk of injury.

On the following pages are suggestions for exercises for the wrist, which can be done both as rehabilitation and as strength training. After all, rehabilitation is simply training while injured, and you can easily control the load based on symptom development during and after training.

If the stabilising structures on the ulnar side of the wrist are injured, it may be advisable to use a brace or orthosis. This can provide a sense of improved stability, and give you confidence to expose the wrist to heavier loads and more demanding movements.

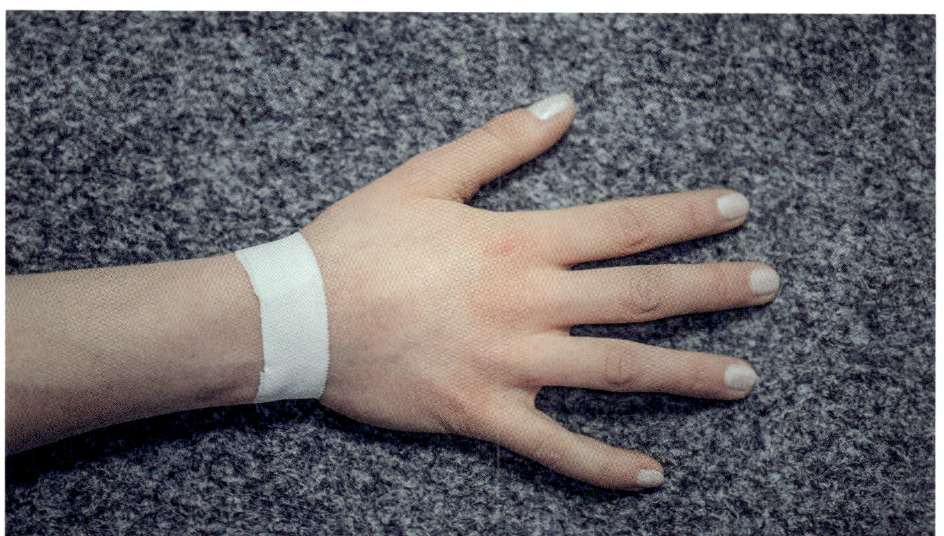

A simple technique to support the wrist on the pinky finger side is to apply circular tape around the wrist.

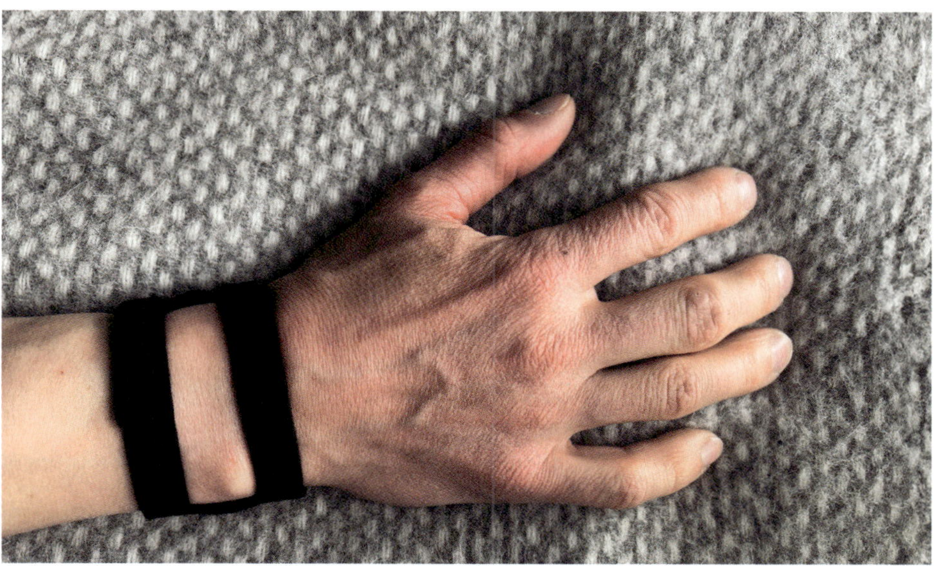

An orthosis (called a WristWidget®) specifically designed to support the TFCC.

EXERCISES

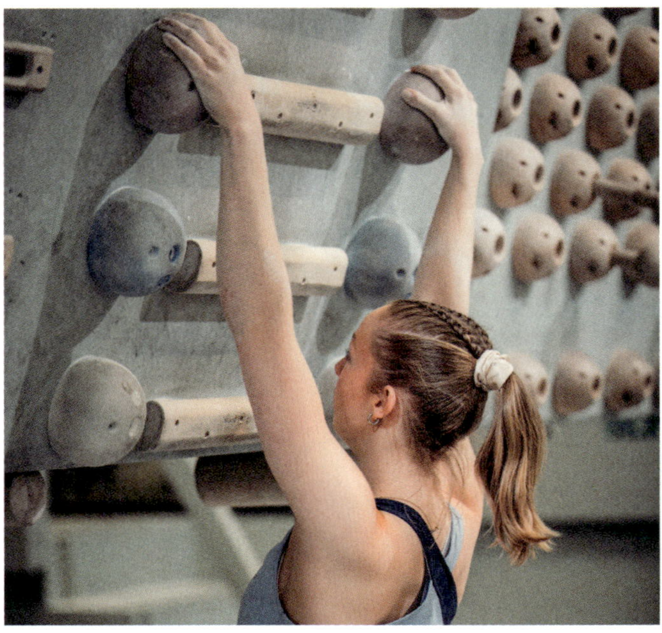

PRACTISE HANGING FROM SLOPERS. As with deadhanging on edges, you can easily control the load by adding to or subtracting from your body weight and adjusting the hang time. To warm up, you can hang for 7–10 seconds, rest for 5 seconds and repeat 5–10 times. For strength training, follow the same progression ladder as for deadhangs on edges (see pages 49–51).

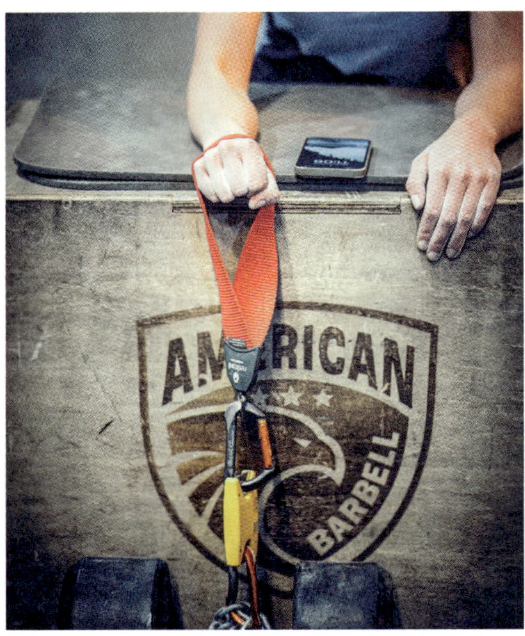

Overcoming isometrics can also be used as a strength training exercise for wrist extension. Use a dumb-bell and place a wide sling over the back of your hand. Push your hand up as hard as you can and hold for 5 seconds. Rest for 1 minute and repeat for 5 sets. If it's painful, you can reduce the force and increase the holding time to 10–15 seconds.

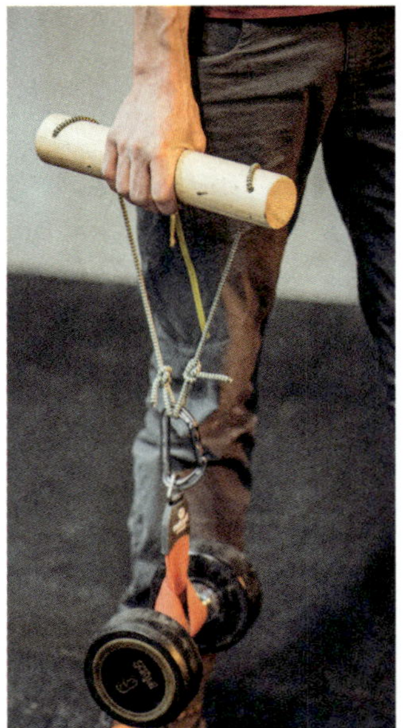

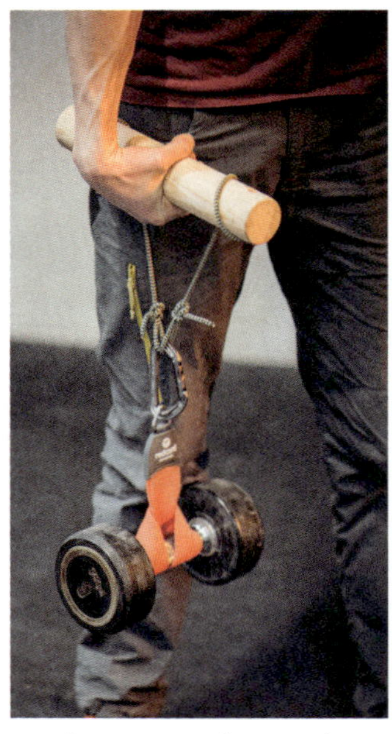

To train wrist flexion in an open grip position, the wrist wrench is a good exercise. Use a wide cylinder (>5cm in diameter) and flex your wrist inwards. Repeat 6–8 times for 3 sets.

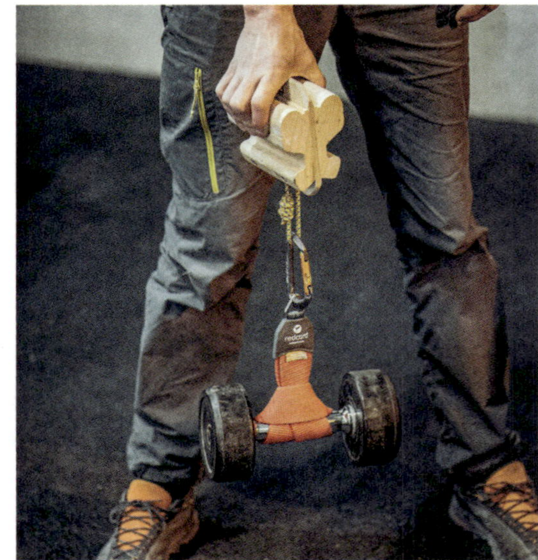

PICK-UP WITH PINCH BLOCK. Start with a weight that you can hold for no more than 10 seconds. Repeat 5 sets with 1–2 minutes' rest in between. Gradually increase the weight and reduce the holding time to 5 seconds per lift.

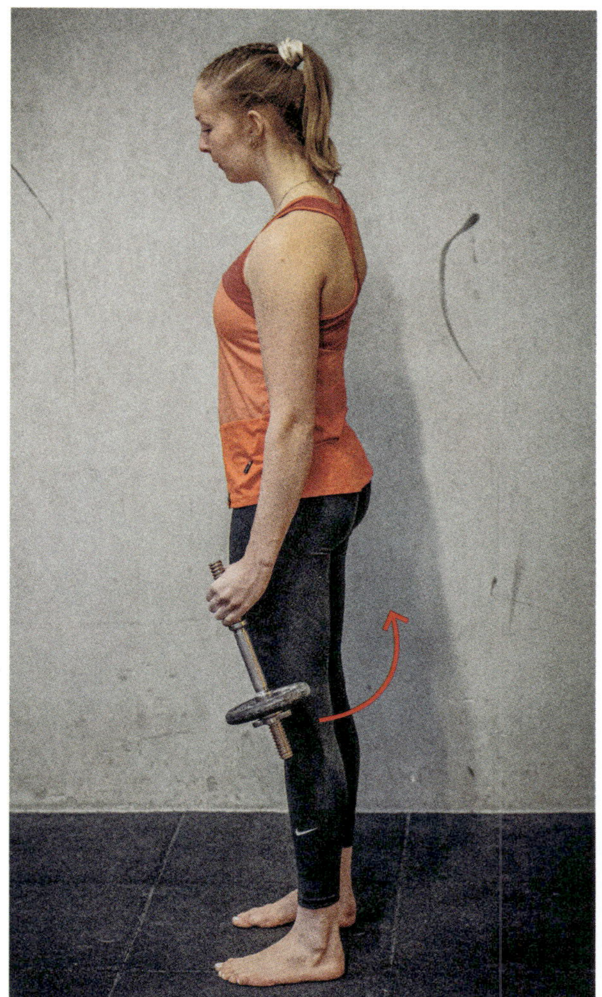

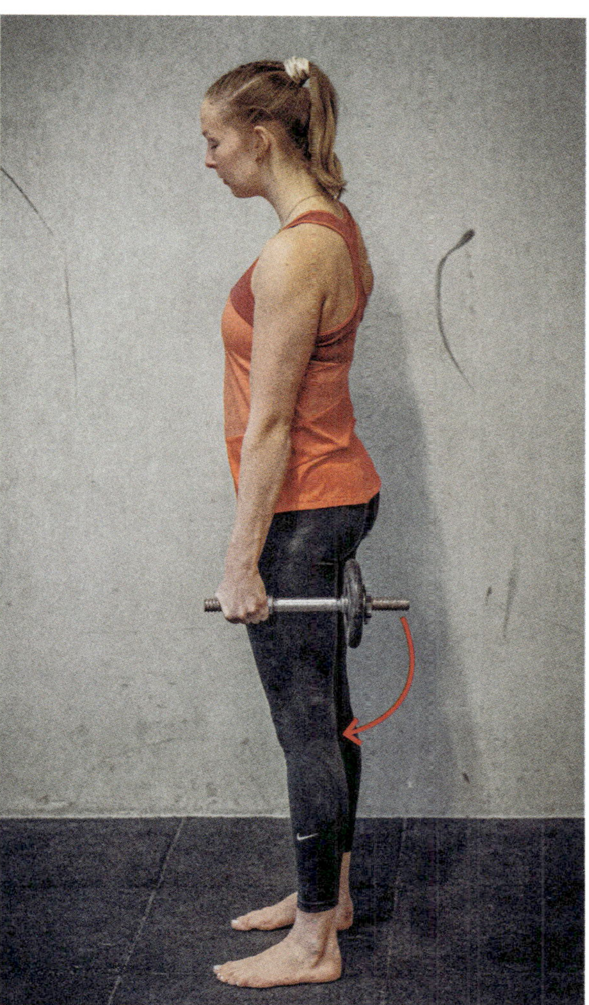

ULNAR FLEXION. In some cases you will want to load into ulnar flexion to strengthen this wrist position. Use a dumb-bell with a disc at one end and lift the weight as shown. Perform 6–8 repetitions for 3 sets.

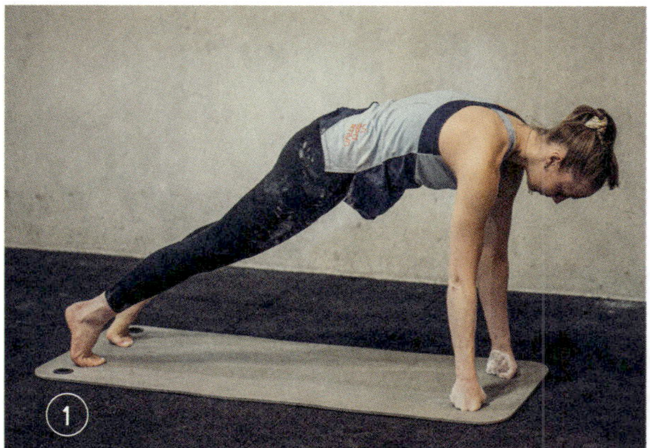

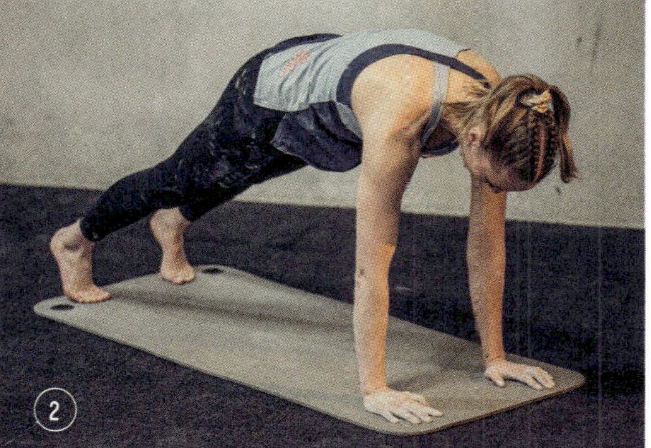

By putting weight on the wrist in small doses, you can gradually regain weight-bearing capacity. Start with your wrist in a neutral position (figure 1) by using your knuckles, then move to weight bearing on your palms (figure 2). Alternate between these positions as part of your warm-up, so that you have exercised your wrist for a total of 3–5 minutes per session.

HOOK OF HAMATE FRACTURE

Yes, I know, this was supposed to be a book about *common* injuries, and this injury is far from common! But it is very specific to climbing, and it is easy to overlook. I have missed it myself, and, unfortunately, it led to a longer rehabilitation than necessary for the unlucky climber. So, consider this an attempt to make up for that oversight, so that this injury is on your radar should it happen to you.

One of the carpal bones is called the *os hamatum*, and it has a hook that stabilises the flexor tendons of the ring and pinky fingers. The English name for this is the *hook of hamate*, and although the most common mechanism of injury is a direct trauma to the inside of the hand, the hook can actually break off from the rest of the bone through intense pressure from these two tendons. This occurs when you flex your wrist towards the pinky side and pull hard with the ring and pinky fingers. In climbing, typical examples are when using undercuts and sidepulls. The injury usually occurs acutely but can also result from repetitive stress over time. The pain is felt deep in the palm, usually a little closer to the pinky side than the thumb side. If there is tenderness when pressure is applied to the area, and a recognisable pain when the ring and pinky fingers are loaded, at least suspect this injury and request an MRI or CT scan. In the case of a fracture, the hand should be immobilised with a cast or support until it can be seen that the hook has fused firmly to the rest of the bone. This should be followed by a rehabilitation period, gradually increasing load while being aware of grip positions. Done properly, you will end up with a fully healed fracture that can withstand higher forces than before the injury. Failed healing might result in a dislocated fracture – meaning that the loose hook does not reattach itself to the rest of bone. In such cases, surgery becomes necessary, but if the injury is caught early on, few will need surgical intervention.

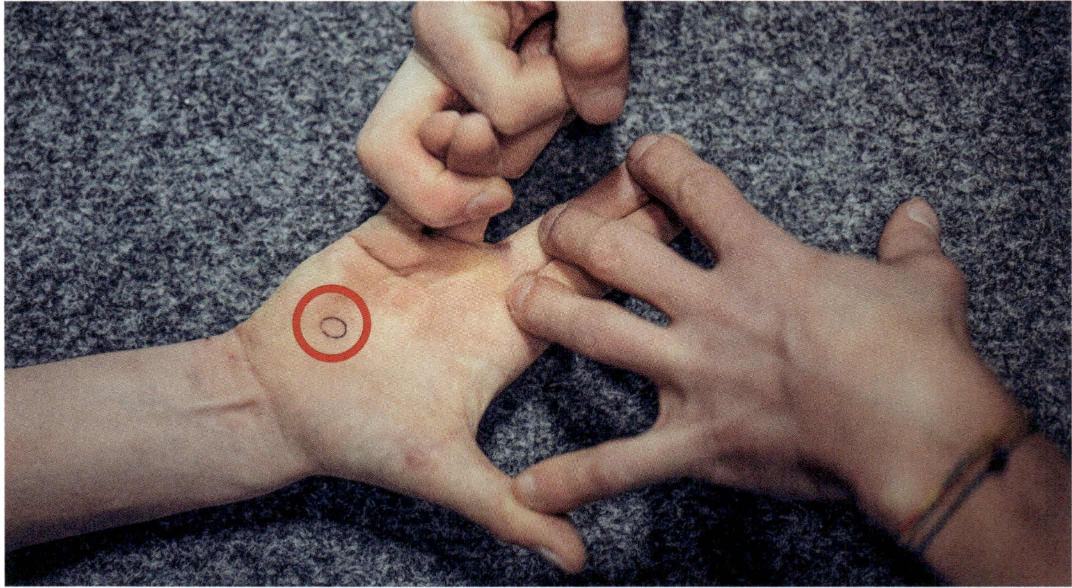

Hook of hamate tension test. Bend your wrist slightly upwards and towards your pinky finger. Then pull hard with your ring and little fingers, putting stress on the hook of hamate, which stabilises the flexor tendons of these two fingers. If there is pain in the area highlighted in the photo above, the hook may be damaged and you should seek a referral for an MRI or CT scan.

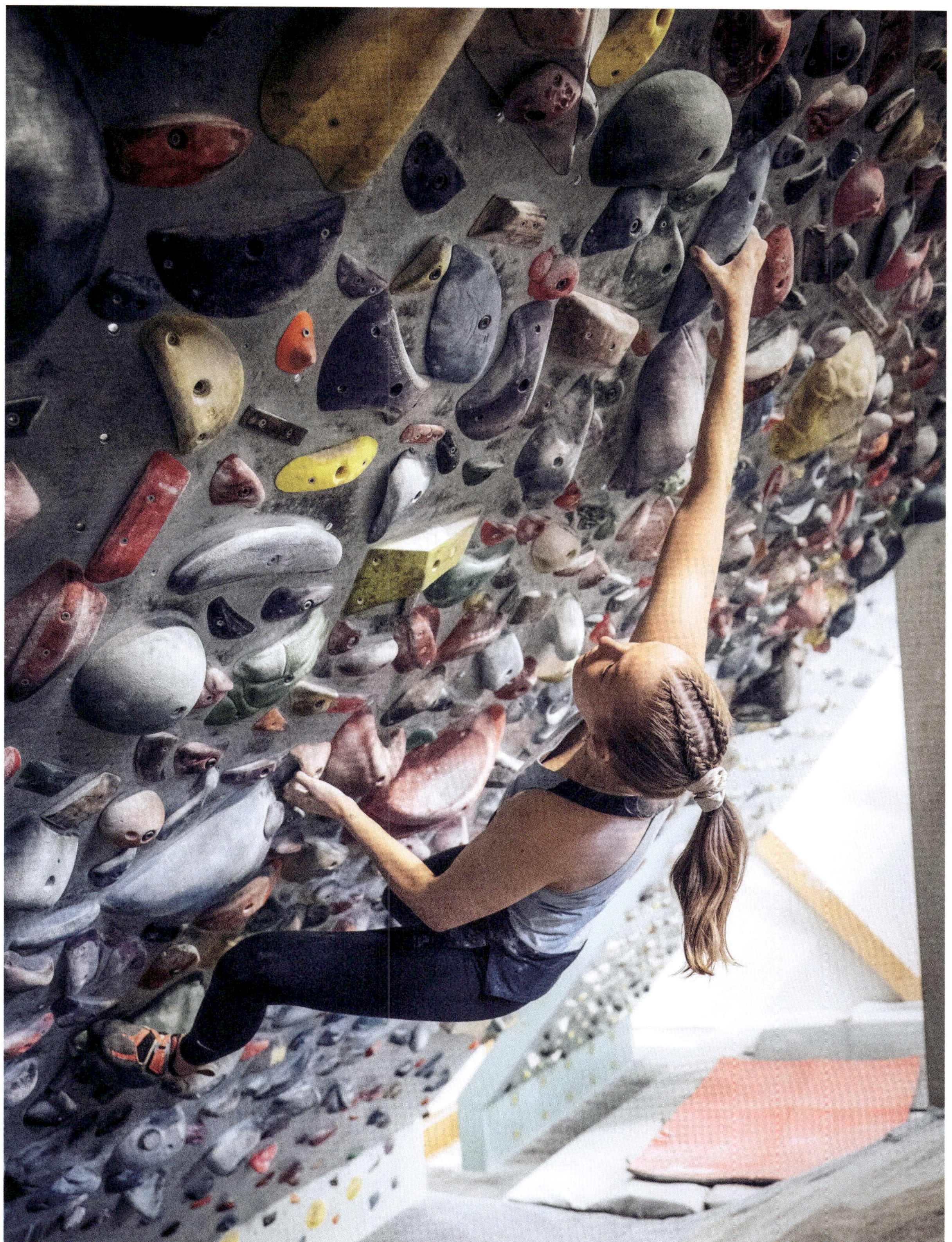

High stress in undercuts, where the wrist is angled towards the pinky finger side, is the most common mechanism cf injury

ELBOWS AND FOREARMS

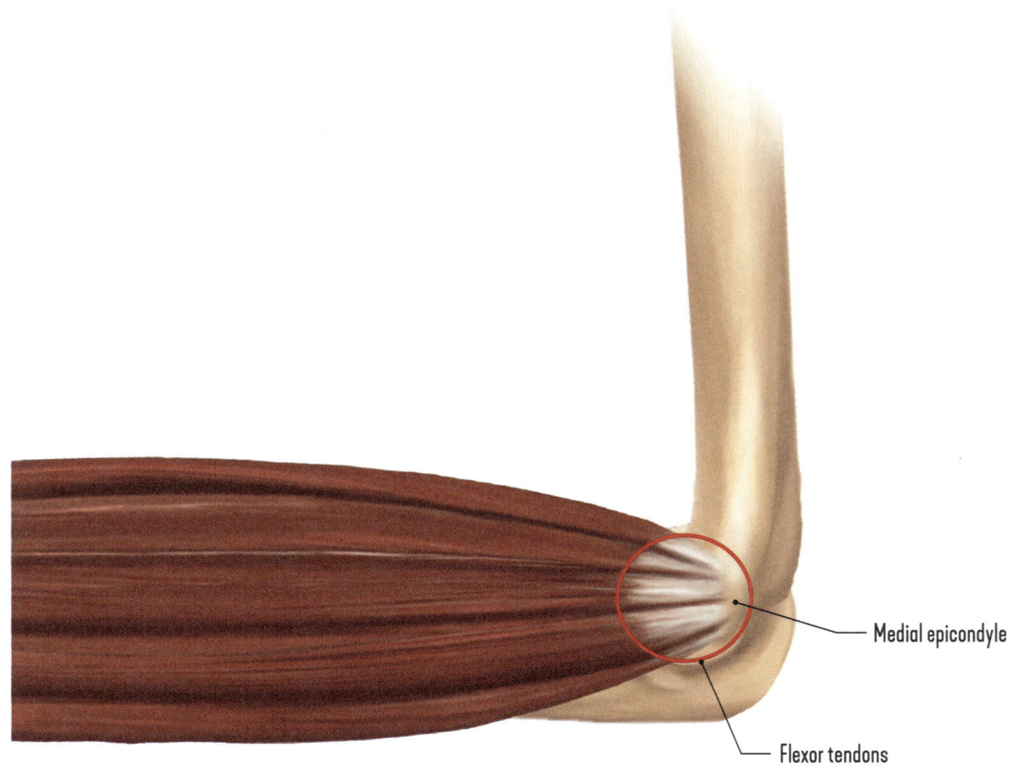

Injuries and pain related to the elbows and forearms are mostly caused by excessive stress over time. However, the elbow is also prone to acute injuries from falls, especially during bouldering. Acute traumatic elbow injuries should always be evaluated by a healthcare professional to detect possible fractures and ligament damage; these injuries are not covered here. This section describes load-related issues related to the forearm muscles and their tendon origins on the inside and outside of the elbow, and pain in the middle aspect of the elbow.

MEDIAL EPICONDYLALGIA – AKA 'GOLFER'S ELBOW'

'It hurts when I press here, on the knuckle on the inside of my elbow. It's painful when I warm up, but climbing can be fine. I notice that it gets worse after climbing, and then it hurts if I slice bread or twist bottle caps.'

The 'knuckle' referred to here is the bony protrusion on the inside – medial side – of the elbow. The knuckle is called the medial epicondyle, so medial epicondylalgia simply refers to pain in this area. The condition is also known as 'golfer's elbow', although a quick Google search shows that it is now also referred to as 'climber's elbow'; however, since this name is reserved for another condition (see page 96), we will stick with golfer's elbow or medial epicondylalgia.

The common tendon for most of the muscles that flex the fingers and wrist and rotate the forearm so that the palm faces downwards (pronation), originates from the medial epicondyle, and the pain primarily relates to reactions in this tendon. The tendon can react due to excessive strain within a short period, but it is also subject to compression forces where it spreads out over the knuckle – particularly when we fully flex our elbows when locking off. Imagine what happens during a pull-up: we grip a bar with our palms facing away from us (a pronated position), using both the flexor muscles of the fingers and wrist and the pronator teres muscle while pulling up into a fully flexed elbow position. If we combine these forces of tension and compression, along with numerous repetitions, the tendon can react and cause pain. Similarly, a high climbing volume on steep or vertical terrain can cause excessive strain, leading to a negative reaction in the tendon.

Although the reaction is a result of doing too much, the solution is not to avoid loading the tendon but rather to break the load down into different components and train them separately.

It is important to emphasise that there is no perfect protocol or training method; instead, we must rely on some basic principles of loading and adaptation in tendon tissue. This provides us with ample opportunities to customise load management in climbing, exercise selection and dosage according to what suits the individual concerned.

Once you experience pain on the insides of your elbows, it's natural to want to climb easier routes or boulders. Although this may seem rational, it is not necessarily the best strategy because most people will climb more when they climb easier. Therefore, the volume increases, and even if you don't climb as hard, the increased volume itself can greatly provoke the tendon. This particularly applies to climbing that is steeper than vertical, since the flexor muscles still have to work relatively hard. Therefore, if you want to climb easier stuff for a while, it is recommended to climb on less steep wall angles and focus on technical elements such as foot placements, balance and weight transfer.

However, it is not necessary to reduce climbing intensity – it is simply the volume that must be reduced. This means shorter sessions, fewer attempts and fewer moves per session, but there's nothing wrong with climbing hard and steep routes or boulders. I have already explained on the previous page why you should avoid deep lock-offs, and although you may find that individual moves can have a negative impact, you can then choose a different boulder or route. The most important thing is still to manage training load according to the so-called '24-hour response' – where the symptoms you experience after a session return to baseline within approximately 24 hours (see page 93).

The principle for effectively managing tendon-related issues is to **load the tendon**, and it is crucial to recognise the possibilities this provides. There is a lot you can do even if your elbow is bothering you, and your goal should be to return as a better and stronger climber. You can achieve this by training technique, doing shorter sessions and working on both finger strength and overall upper-body strength – there is significantly more you can do than what you need to avoid. There are numerous examples of high-level climbers who have climbed hard routes and boulders despite dealing with golfer's elbow. They were able to accomplish this by being aware of which moves and types of climbing worsened their symptoms, so that they could choose different routes and boulders. This approach, combined with the fact that this condition *will* improve over time, is sufficient in most cases. However, there are exercises you can try if you want to be more specific in your approach.

Unfortunately, golfer's elbow tends to cause symptoms for several months and tends to flare up again when you exceed the limit of how much load the elbow can handle. It is important to be aware that this is a natural part of the process and you should use the symptoms as a tool to choose exercises, types of workouts and training methods. Through a combination of load management while climbing and doing specific strength training, you can effectively manage the condition until it eventually disappears.

EXERCISES

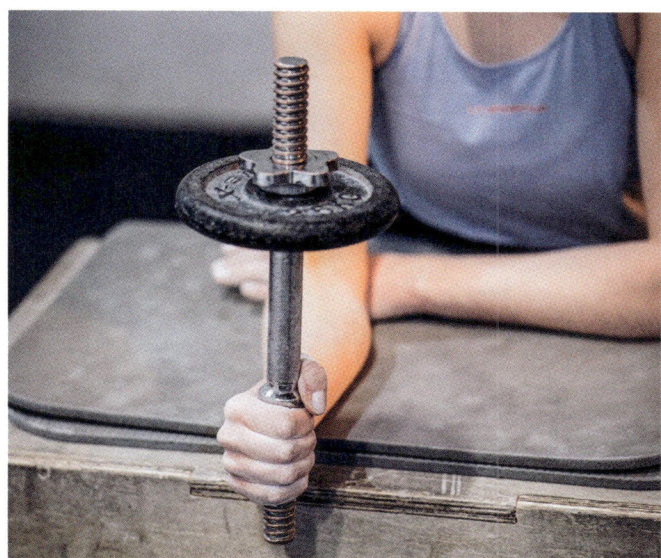

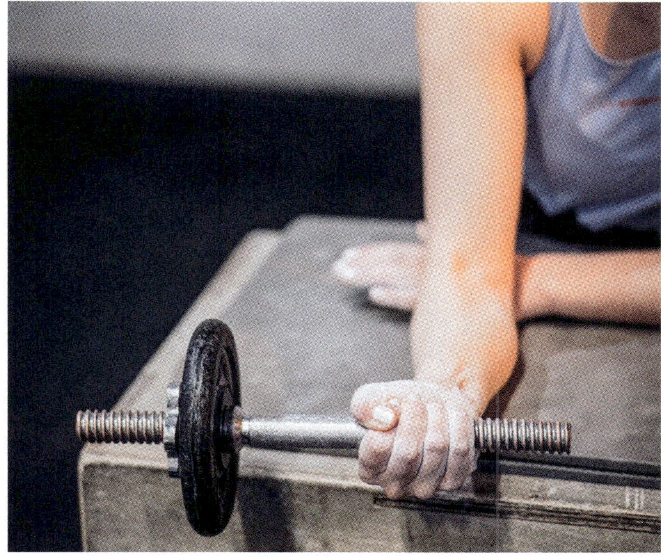

PRONATION AND SUPINATION. Using a dumb-bell with a weight disc at one end, start with the weight facing up and slowly lower it out to the side before returning to the starting position. Start with a weight that does not cause unacceptable pain and aim for 10–12 repetitions. Initially, you can do one such set every day, then increase the weight, reduce the number of repetitions, increase the number of sets per session and do only 1–2 such sessions a week. It may then look like this: 4–6 repetitions in 3–4 sets, 1–2 times a week.

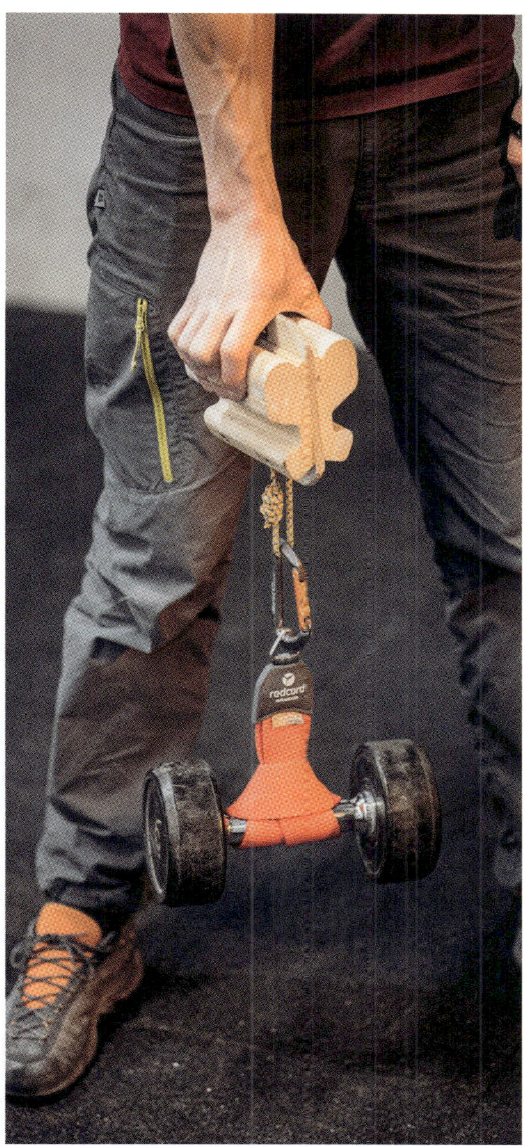

PICK-UP WITH PINCH BLOCK. Start with a weight that you can hold for no more than 10 seconds. Repeat for 5 sets with 1–2 minutes' rest in between. Gradually increase the weight and reduce the holding time to 3–5 seconds per lift. Then do 4 lifts of 3–5 seconds with a 5-second rest in between and repeat for 4 sets.

EXERCISES

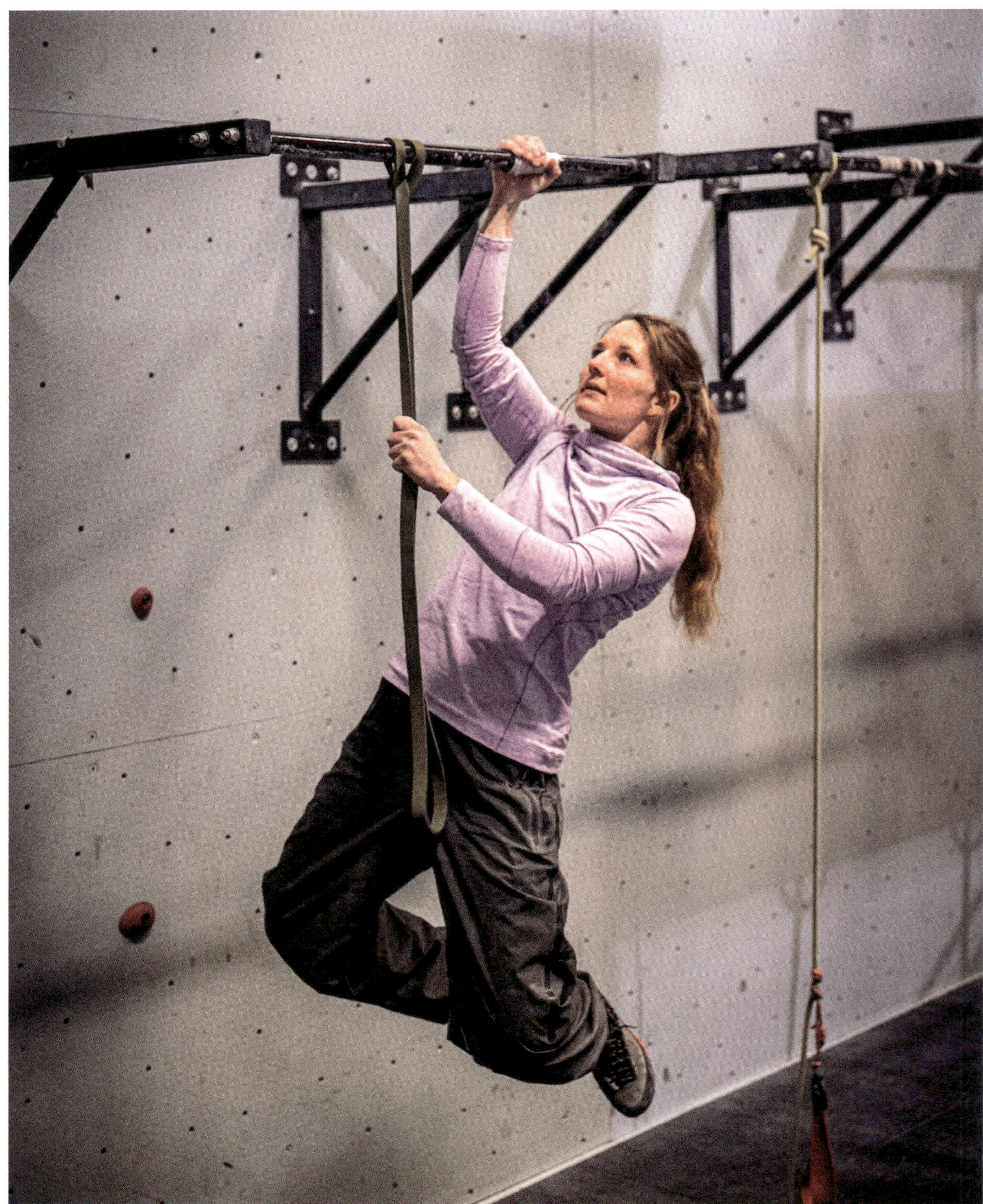

ONE-ARM LOCK-OFF. You can either reduce your body weight or add extra weight to find the right load for you. Aim for a hang time of 10 seconds as a starting point and reduce the hang time to 5 seconds as you increase the weight. Repeat in 3–4 sets with 1–2 minutes' rest.

LOCK-OFF ON TWO ARMS and **DEADHANG** are good starting points for long hang times, i.e. hang times of up to 25–30 seconds. Isometric loading with a long time under tension means that forces within the tendon are reduced, allowing us to address the part of the tendon that is shielded. This shielding is called 'stress shielding' and is a mechanism to prevent further damage to the tendon tissue. You can start with a 15-second hang and gradually increase to 30 seconds and do 2 sets of lock-offs and 2 sets of deadhangs.

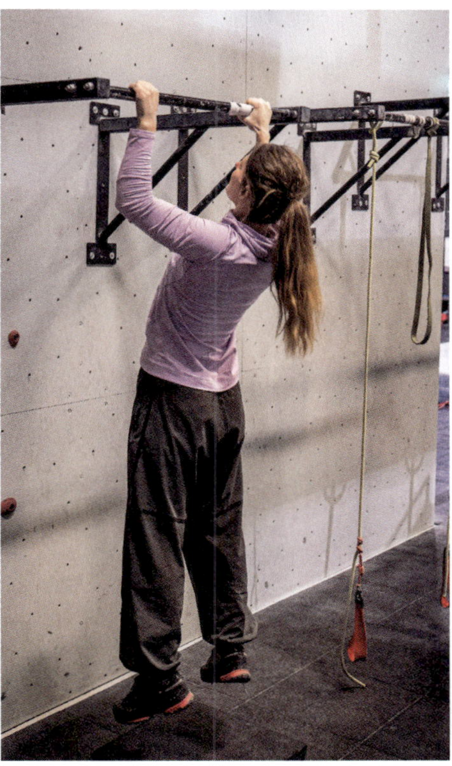

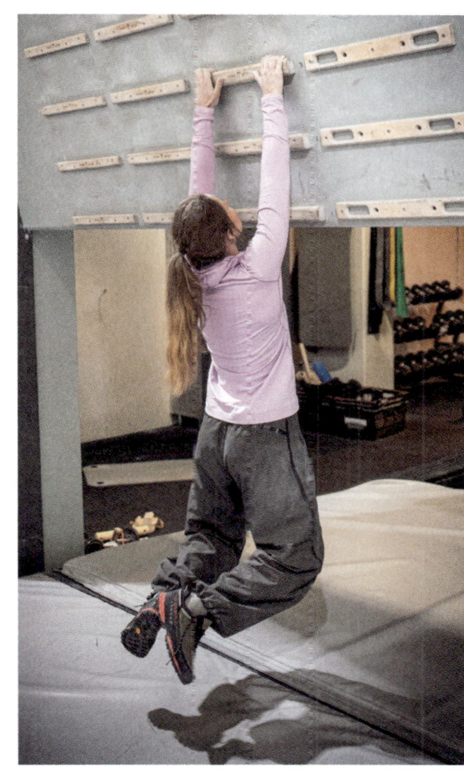

JUMP-START. At the opposite end of the scale from 'stress shielding' and 'stress relaxation' are training methods that stimulate stiffness in the tendon tissue and improve the tendon's ability to store and release elastic energy. An example of a training method for these properties is jump-starts, where the focus is on landing the top hold. You can do 4–8 such jumps per arm and repeat for 3 sets.

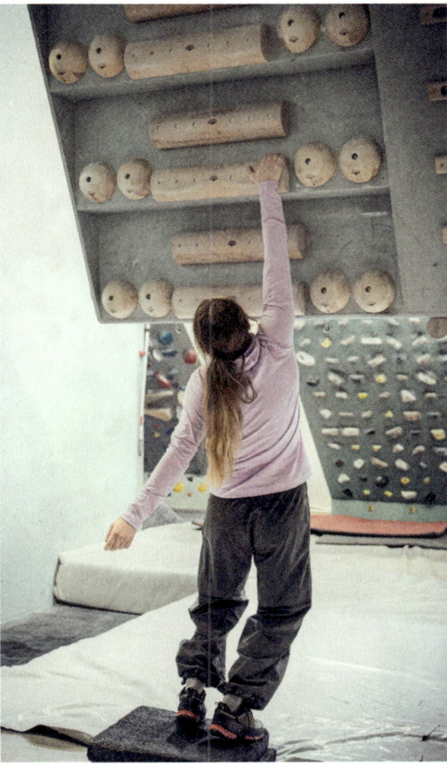

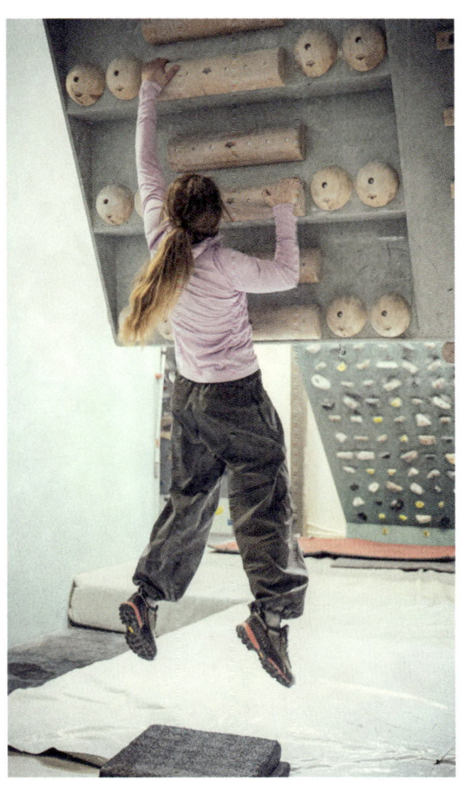

TENDINOPATHY

Changes in tendon tissue can occur as a natural part of the ageing process, or as a reaction to both excessive and insufficient load. These changes result in reduced tendon fibre quality and an ingrowth of blood vessels and nerve endings into the tendon tissue. However, such changes to the tendon are also seen in people without symptoms, and it is only when there are both tissue changes *and* pain during loading of the tendon that we call it *tendinopathy*. This term has replaced the previous term 'tendonitis', where 'itis' refers to an inflammation that we currently have difficulties identifying. Calling such tendon-related problems inflammations is incorrect, and measures aimed at reducing an inflammatory response – such as rest, cooling and anti-inflammatory medication – will not have the desired effect.

What is important for our purposes is that **tendons adapt to load by being loaded**. There are many ways to load tendon tissue, but since load is crucial for both resolving symptoms and increasing the capacity of the tendon to handle load, complete rest is rarely a good option. Australian tendon researcher Jill Cook has proposed a progression model for tendinopathies, which serves as a good framework for adapting exercises, load and activities. By following such a progression model, we can always adjust the load based on symptom response and gradually build up the capacity to tolerate whatever we expose our tendons to.

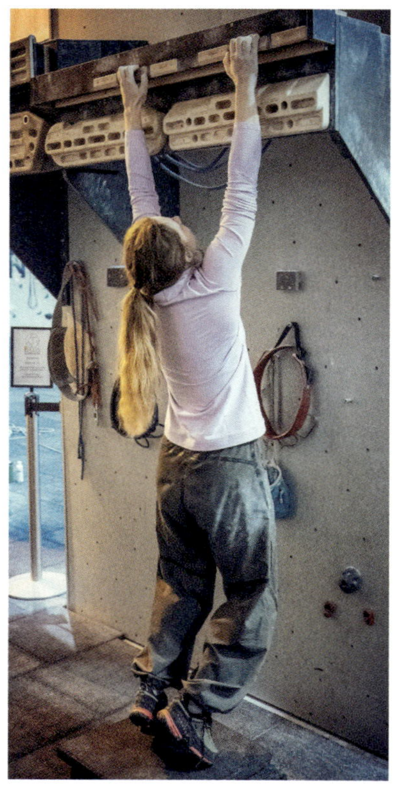

NO-HANG. 10 seconds on/30 seconds off x10 in different grip positions. This will work all the muscle-tendon units involved in a grip position, including the tendons in the elbow.

As an addition to this model, it should be noted that short sessions done frequently are suggested as a method to stimulate the tendon cells. As little as 10 minutes of low-load exercise stimulates the cells to produce more collagen tissue, which is beneficial for a tendinopathic tendon. After a session, it takes about six hours for the cells to become responsive to load again, so a protocol early in rehabilitation could be one short session three times a day with six hours' rest between each session.

One way to do this is through so-called *no-hangs*, where you can load for 10 seconds, rest for 30 seconds and do 10–20 repetitions.* The load should be low, preferably down to 30 per cent of 1RM (one repetition maximum), and the aim is not to tire the muscles.

Further training of the tendon should mainly focus on progressively heavier loads, since mechanical tension is what makes the tendon stronger and stiffer. A proposed protocol to stimulate this is 3 seconds' effort, followed by 3 seconds' rest, x4 repetitions, x5 sets, where the intensity in each repetition is over 90 per cent of 1RM. This can easily be done as isometric training on a fingerboard, using a grip tool or with weights depending on which tendons you primarily want to target.

To supplement this 'heavy loading' regime, you can expose the tendon to energy storage and release. This includes reducing the mechanical load but increasing the velocity and/or rate of force development. Following these principles, you'll build up the muscle-tendon unit to its previous capacity – and beyond.

*No-hang means, as the name suggests, that you are not hanging from the edges but standing on the ground and pressing your fingertips against the grip surface, whether it is a fingerboard or a portable grip tool.

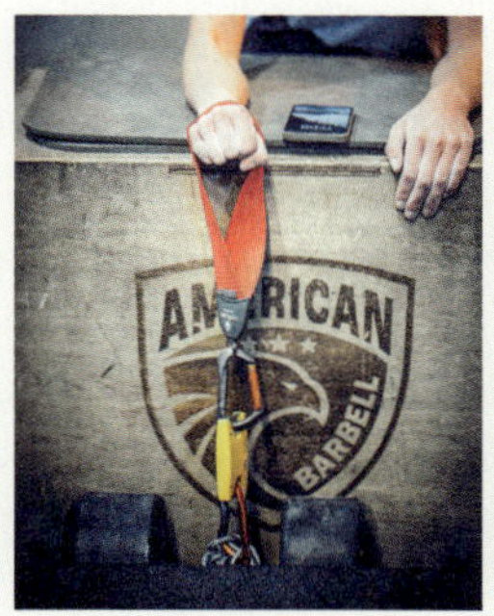

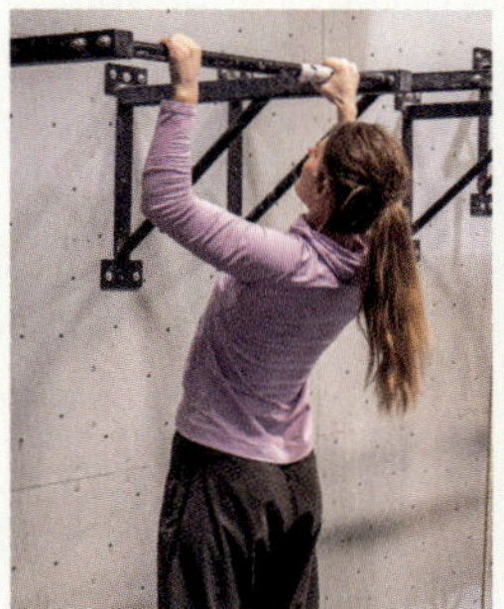

STEP 1:
Isometric training without compression.

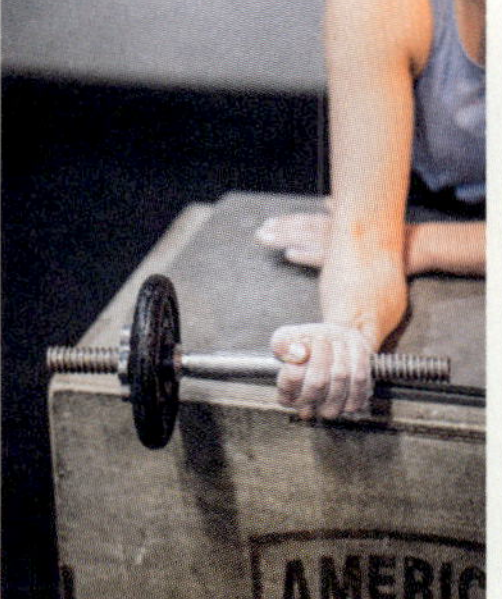

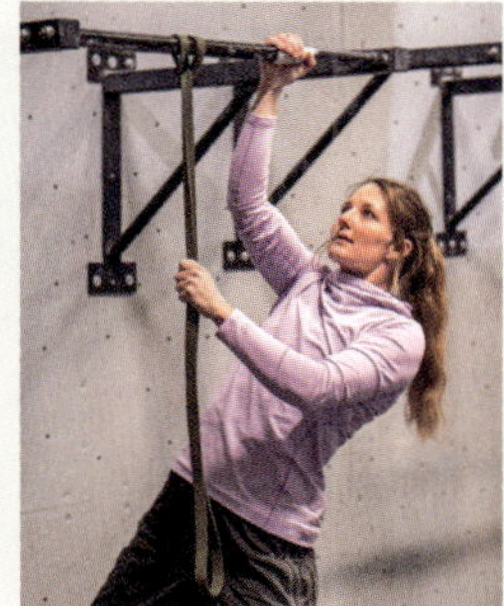

STEP 2:
Strength, without compression. Kinetic chain, functional for the activity.

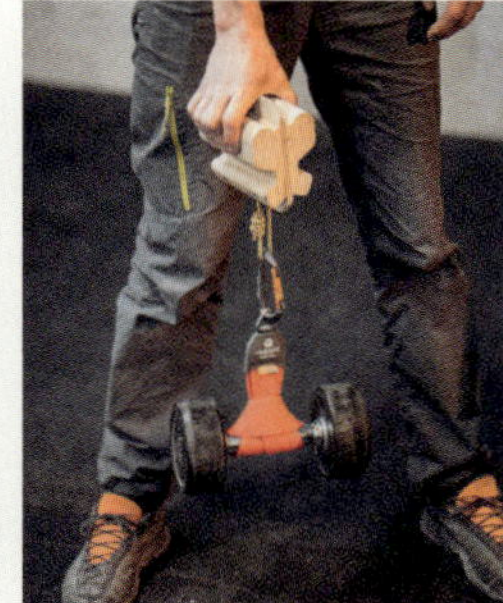

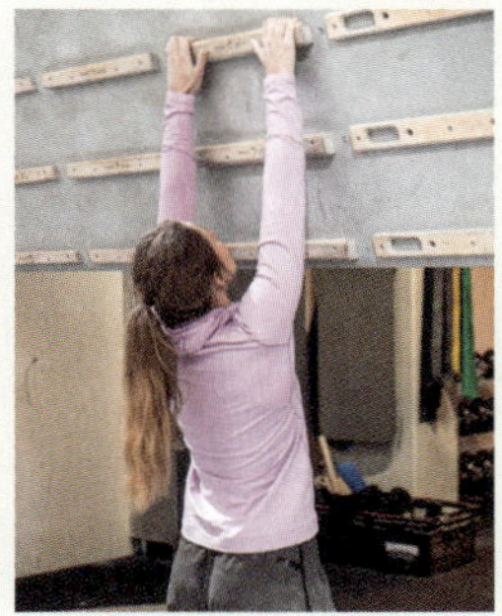

STEP 3:
Energy storage. Faster movements. Eccentric in the outer position. Exercises at a faster pace.

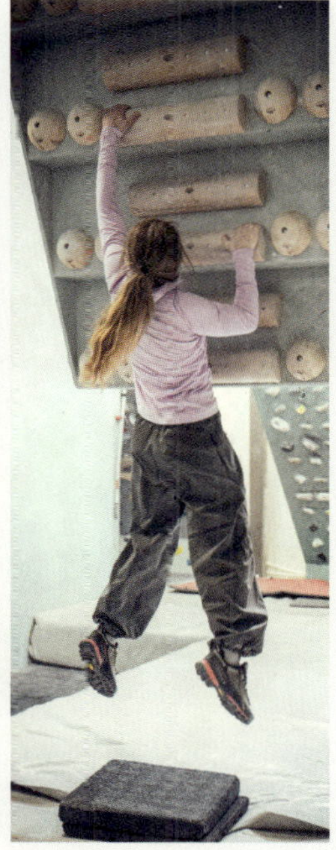

STEP 4:
Energy storage and release, stretch-shorten-cycle (SSC). No restrictions, sport specific.

Both the no-hang and heavy load protocols can be used for different specific exercises, aiming to create mechanical tension which again stimulates adaptation in the tendon tissue. It's therefore possible to combine this training with more functional exercises, which will include far more elements than just adding mechanical tension to the tendon.

24-HOUR RESPONSE

It can be difficult to use pain as an indicator of tissue damage, or as a sign of overdoing things. As we will see later in the book in chapter 3, pain is an experience that is based on far more than tissue damage, yet it is still the symptom we're left with and which we must try to make sense of after exercise. Dealing with this symptom response from a 24-hour perspective makes us less vulnerable to transient changes in pain and allows us to look more towards a trend line that develops over time. Naturally, it can hurt to load a painful body part, and it is likely that a symptom response will be experienced after exercising throughout a rehabilitation process. However, as long as these symptoms return to baseline within 24 hours, we can continue rehabilitation and see that the trend line moves in the right direction – despite transient pain responses along the way.

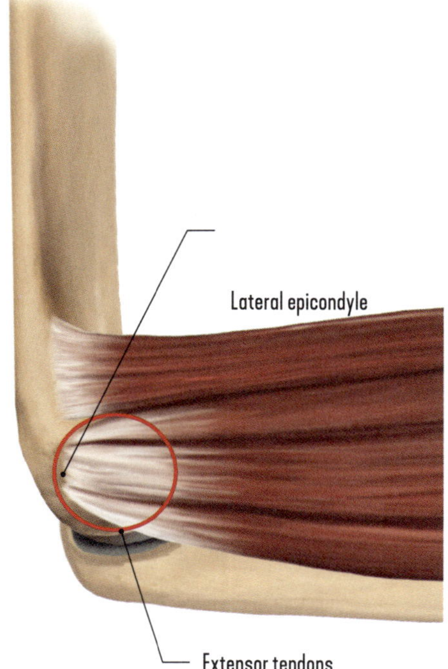

LATERAL EPICONDYLALGIA – AKA 'TENNIS ELBOW'

'It hurts here, over this knuckle. I notice it especially when I take a milk carton from the fridge, or when I unscrew the lid of a jam jar. After climbing, it hurts even more, and my elbow feels stiff when I wake up in the morning.'

The description above is not unlike that of medial epicondylalgia, but this time it concerns the knuckle on the outside – lateral side – of the elbow. Therefore, the condition is called lateral epicondylalgia, but it is better known as 'tennis elbow'. If you're not familiar with tennis, hitting a ball with a racket involves gripping around the racket and angling your wrist backwards during the swing phase. This backward angling is called wrist extension, and the muscle-tendon units that perform this movement originate from the lateral epicondyle. Rather than hitting a ball with a racket, more relevant for us climbers is that we're completely dependent on wrist extension for generating force when gripping. Just try flexing your wrist while loading your fingers in a half-crimp position – you won't be able to generate much force. So, every time we hold on to a grip, we automatically extend our wrists and thus load our extensor muscles along with their associated tendons. We also rely on the extensor muscles in our fingers and wrists to maintain a grip position, and the importance of wrist extension is nicely illustrated through the phenomenon known as 'chicken winging', which occurs when we're pumped.

Tennis elbow is a tendinopathy, just like golfer's elbow, so the principles described on pages 92–93 for how we manage tendinopathies also apply in this case. By adjusting the load (primarily by reducing the volume), avoiding deep lock-offs, supplementing with the exercises on pages 89–91 and then gradually increasing the volume again, we will in most cases be able to train and climb throughout rehab. Despite tennis elbow – like golfer's elbow – being able to cause symptoms for several months, there is still more we can do than we should avoid, and we can control the training load based on the 24-hour response described on page 93.

See exercises on pages 89–91.

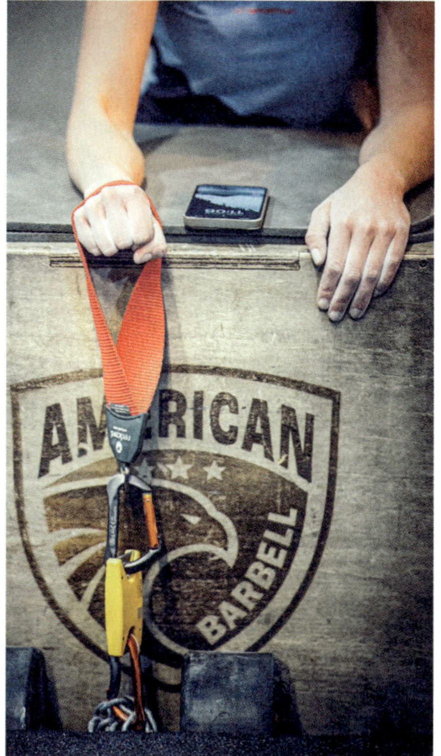

LOAD CELL. Wrist extension provides a direct mechanical pull on the tendon insertion at the lateral epicondyle. By using an isometric training method with a load cell, you can control how much effort you can put in before the pain becomes unacceptable, and you can further control the training by increasing the length of time you hold the position.

CHICKEN WINGING

Have you ever wondered why we climbers raise our elbows when we're getting pumped? This strange phenomenon we call chicken winging is caused by us automatically trying to achieve a better joint angle for the flexor muscles of the fingers. As these muscles tire when climbing, the elbows start to rise and bend backward in relation to the wrists, and it looks like we have chicken wings.

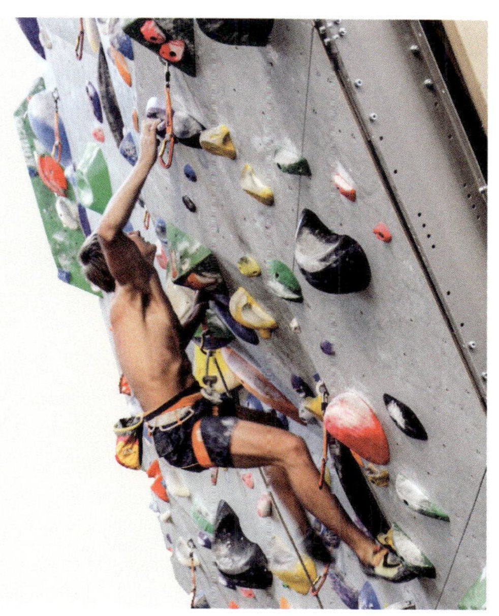

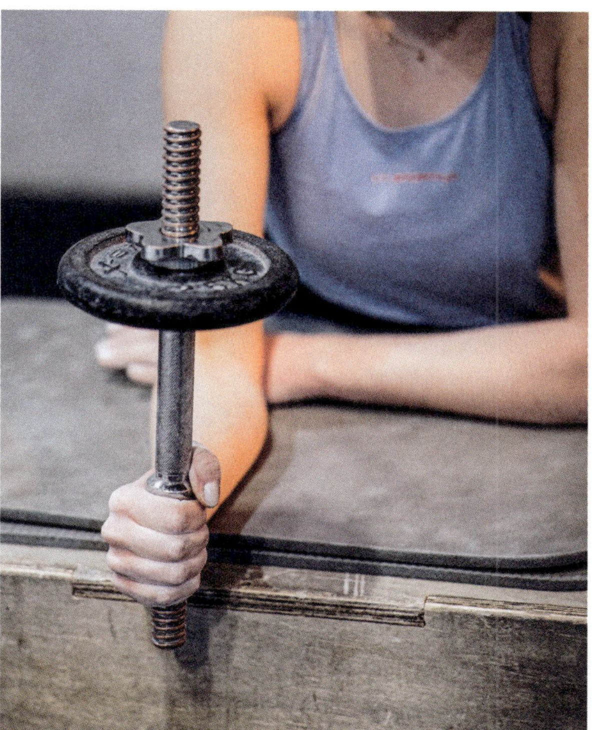

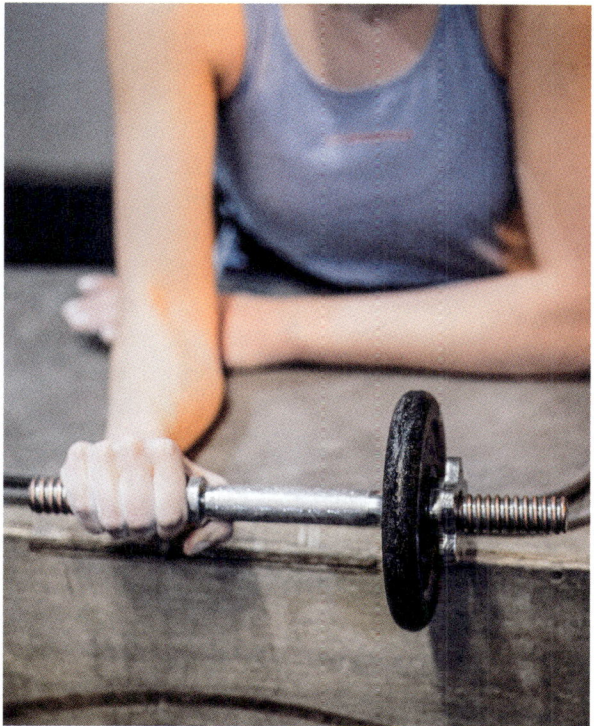

PRONATION AND SUPINATION. Using a dumb-bell with a weight disc at one end, start with the weight pointing upwards and slowly lower it towards the middle before returning to the starting position. Start with a weight that does not cause unacceptable pain and aim for 10–12 repetitions. Initially you can do 1 set a day and then increase the weight, reduce the number of repetitions, increase the number of sets per session and do only 1–2 sets per week. It may then look like this: 4–6 repetitions in 3–4 sets, 1–2 times a week.

CLIMBER'S ELBOW

'It aches here, around the biceps and down to the elbow. It feels sore and stiff and gets much worse after steep climbing or during pull-ups.'

These symptoms, located on the front of the elbow, were described in the literature as far back as 1988 by Bollen, and were then called 'climber's elbow'. The symptoms were associated with pull-up training and traversing, and what these movements have in common is that the forearm is rotated so that the palm faces away from you while the elbow is flexed. With such pronation of the forearm, the biceps muscle is no longer the primary elbow flexor. This causes the brachialis muscle, which lies underneath the biceps and flexes the elbow regardless of the forearm position, to work harder.

Like both golfer's elbow and tennis elbow, this condition can develop into a tendinopathy in the brachialis tendon, but this has not been investigated in research to date. Based on my own experiences with ultrasound scanning, however, it is extremely rare for me to see tendinopathic changes in the tendon itself; therefore, this condition appears to be more related to the muscle than to the tendon. The cause is almost always excessive and repetitive loading over time, including a lot of pull-up training and steep climbing – especially steep compression climbing on sloping holds where we 'slap' on to grips. In addition to the previously mentioned positioning of the forearm, climbing on steep wall angles causes us to work statically with flexed elbows and with rapid transitions between eccentric and concentric phases, where we respectively grip and move on with the opposite arm.

The solution is, of course, to reduce the strain on the brachialis muscles by training at less steep wall angles and stopping pull-up training for a period. This does not mean that you cannot train strength, but that you must adjust the forearm position to neutral or supinated. You can therefore train one-arm lock-offs, with or without assistance, biceps curls and pull-ups with neutral or supinated grip. You can also adjust the wall angle slightly, for example down to 30–40 degrees, and climb on smaller holds with shorter moves; this will put less strain on the brachialis muscles than large moves on bigger holds on steeper terrain.

As with tendinopathies, loading the brachialis muscles is essential in order to return to climbing. Therefore, it is likely that there will be some pain and discomfort associated with training, but as long as you are able to perform the exercises without pain hindering force development, and there is no persistent pain response afterwards, the discomfort during and after training is completely okay. This is a harmless condition that in most cases improves completely just by managing the load and avoiding the worst triggers for a short period of time.

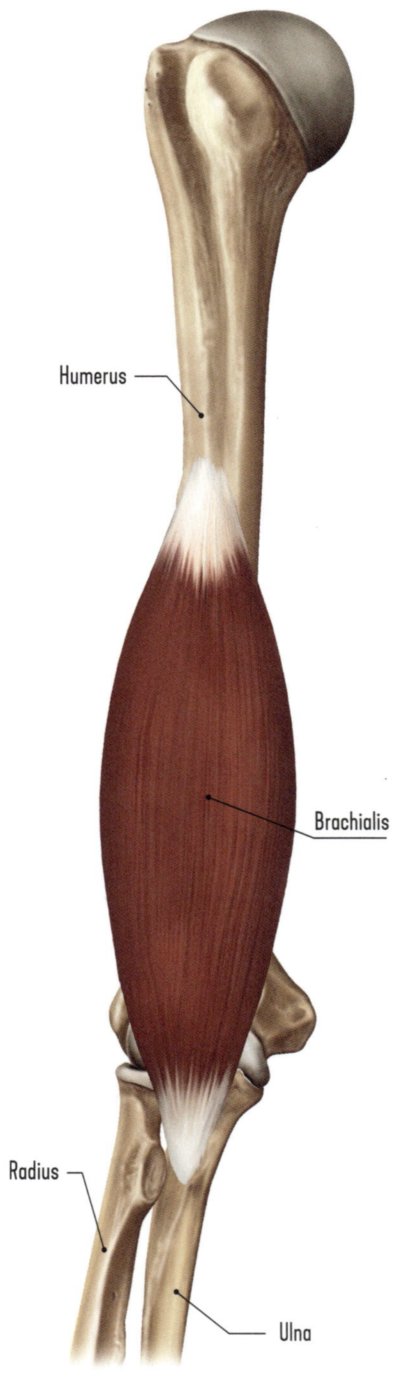

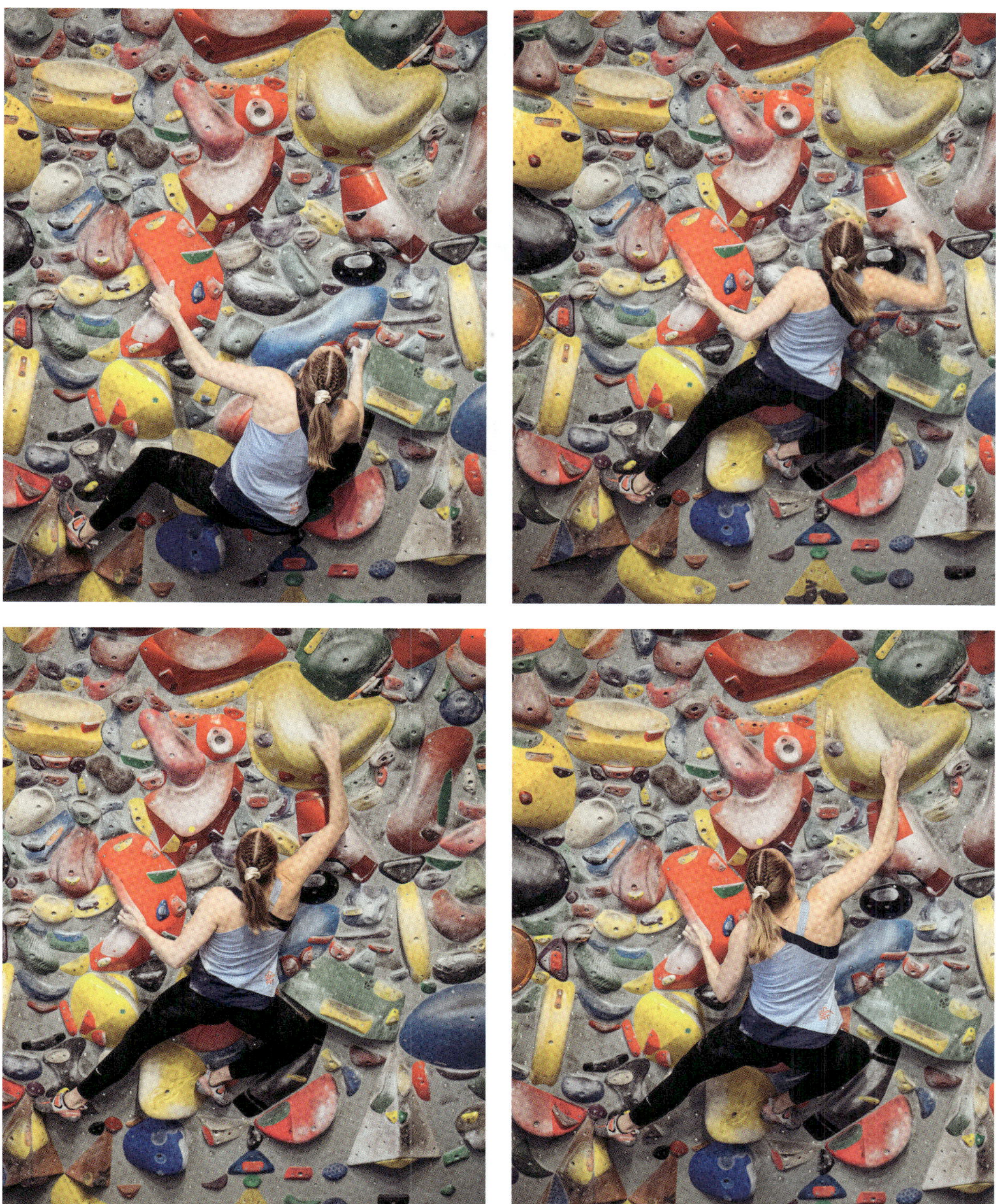

COMPRESSION CLIMBING ON SLOPERS. The body position is maintained by compressing between the holds, i.e. squeezing your arms together. In one movement, you release this tension when you let go with one hand and regain it as quickly as possible when you reach the next hold. This combination of rapid force development, eccentric loading in the landing phase and a long period of brachialis tension is a likely cause of anterior elbow pain.

EXERCISES

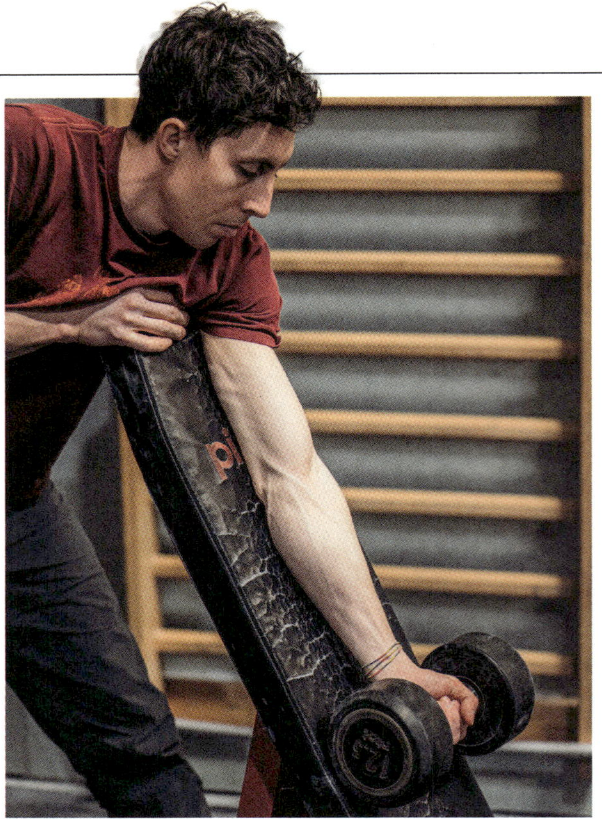

BICEPS CURLS. Place your arm over a bench and start with the elbow straight. Slowly raise the arm and return it to the starting position. In this way, you can work the brachialis muscle hard while it is supported by the biceps muscle. Aim to work as hard as you can for 4–6 repetitions in 2 sets.

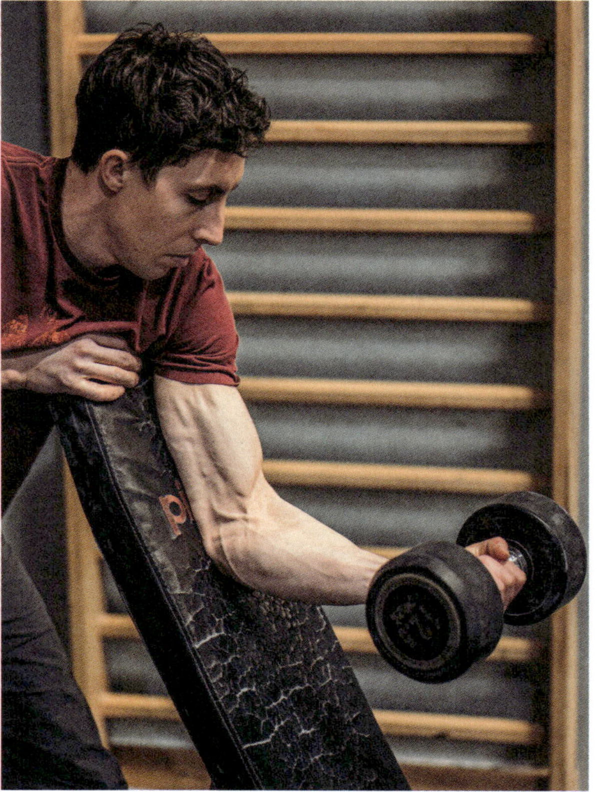

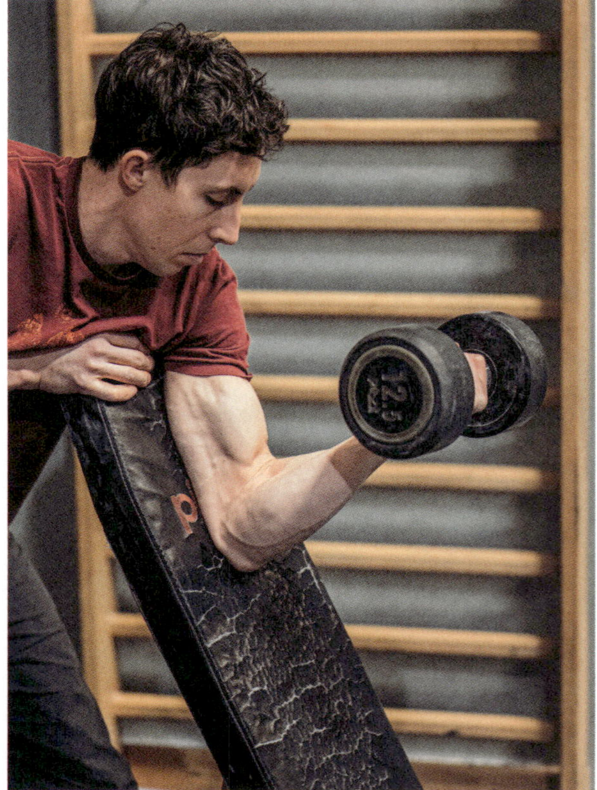

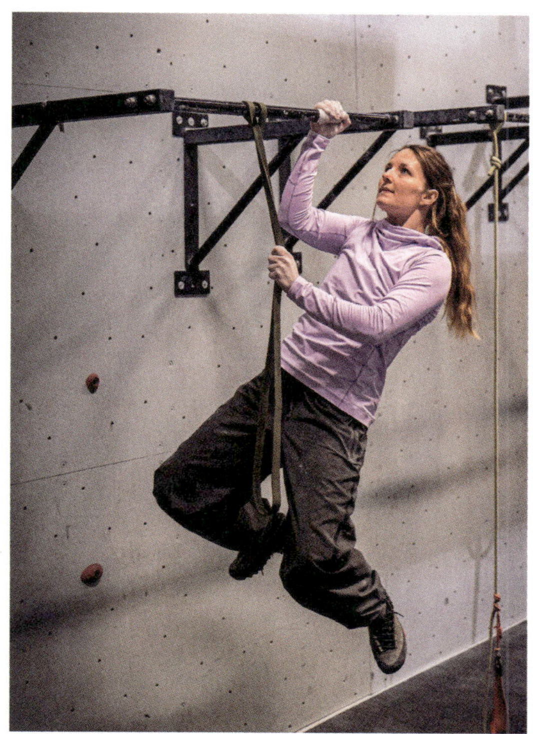

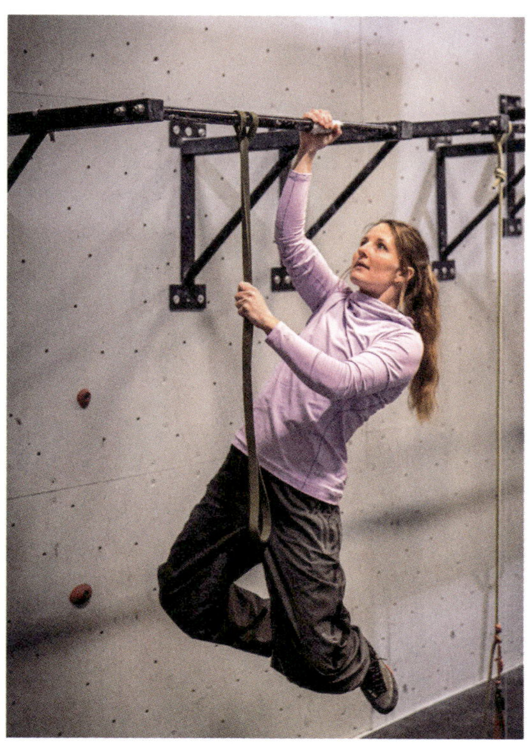

ASSISTED ONE-ARM LOCK-OFFS. Do 2 sets of 10 seconds each, at both 90 degrees and 135 degrees of elbow flexion.

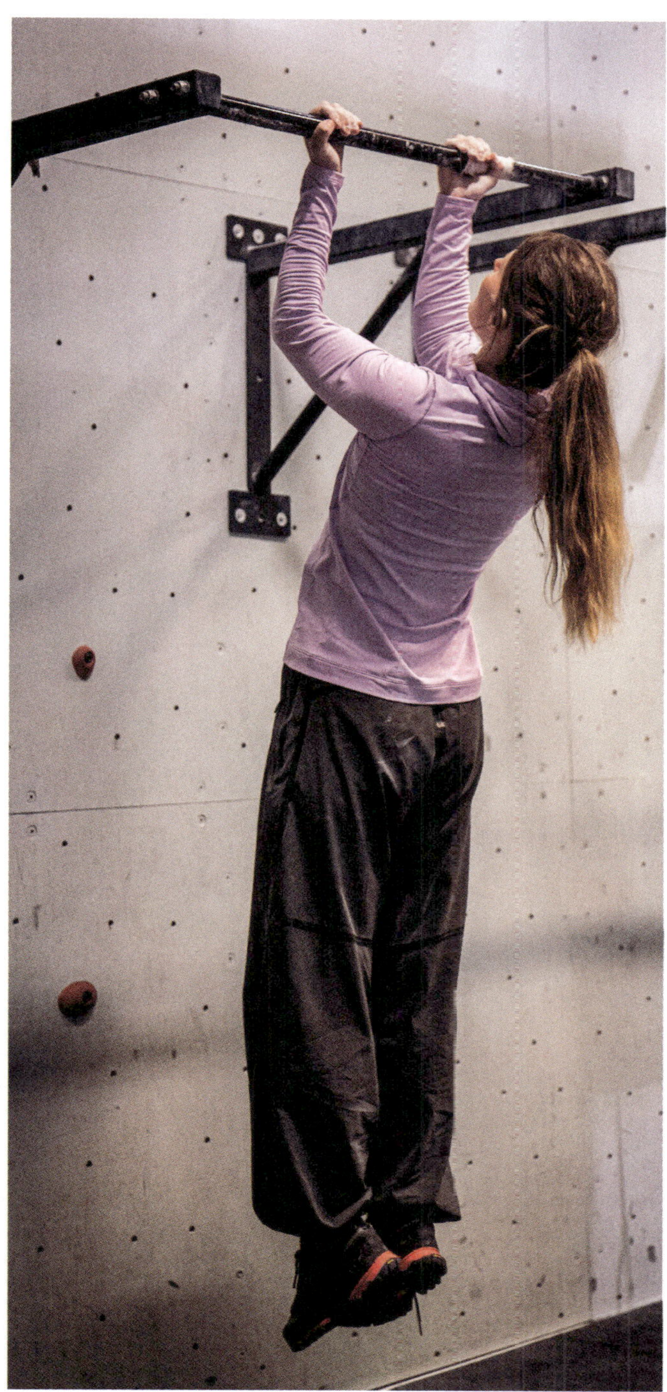

UNDERHAND PULL-UPS (AKA CHIN-UPS). Start with your arms straight and pull up until your chin is over the bar. As with biceps curls, the biceps muscles now assist the brachialis muscles flexing the elbows. Either use bungee cords under your legs for assistance or add extra weight if necessary to complete 4–6 repetitions in 2 sets.

PHOTO: STIAN CHRISTOPHERSEN

FUN FACT

The loading pattern with pronated forearm and repetitive load is commonly seen when bouldering on the sandstone boulders of Fontainebleau in France. Most of the boulders you will find in Font have a rounded top, often with nothing more than pure friction as the only means of topping out. You must then press the palms of your hands down on the holds at the same time as flexing your elbows to pull your body up. This movement pattern is central to almost all of the top-outs, independent of the level of difficulty of the boulder problem, and is repeated every day when you are out climbing in Font. Many climbers end up suffering from climber's elbow when visiting Fontainebleau, hence the nickname 'Font elbow'.

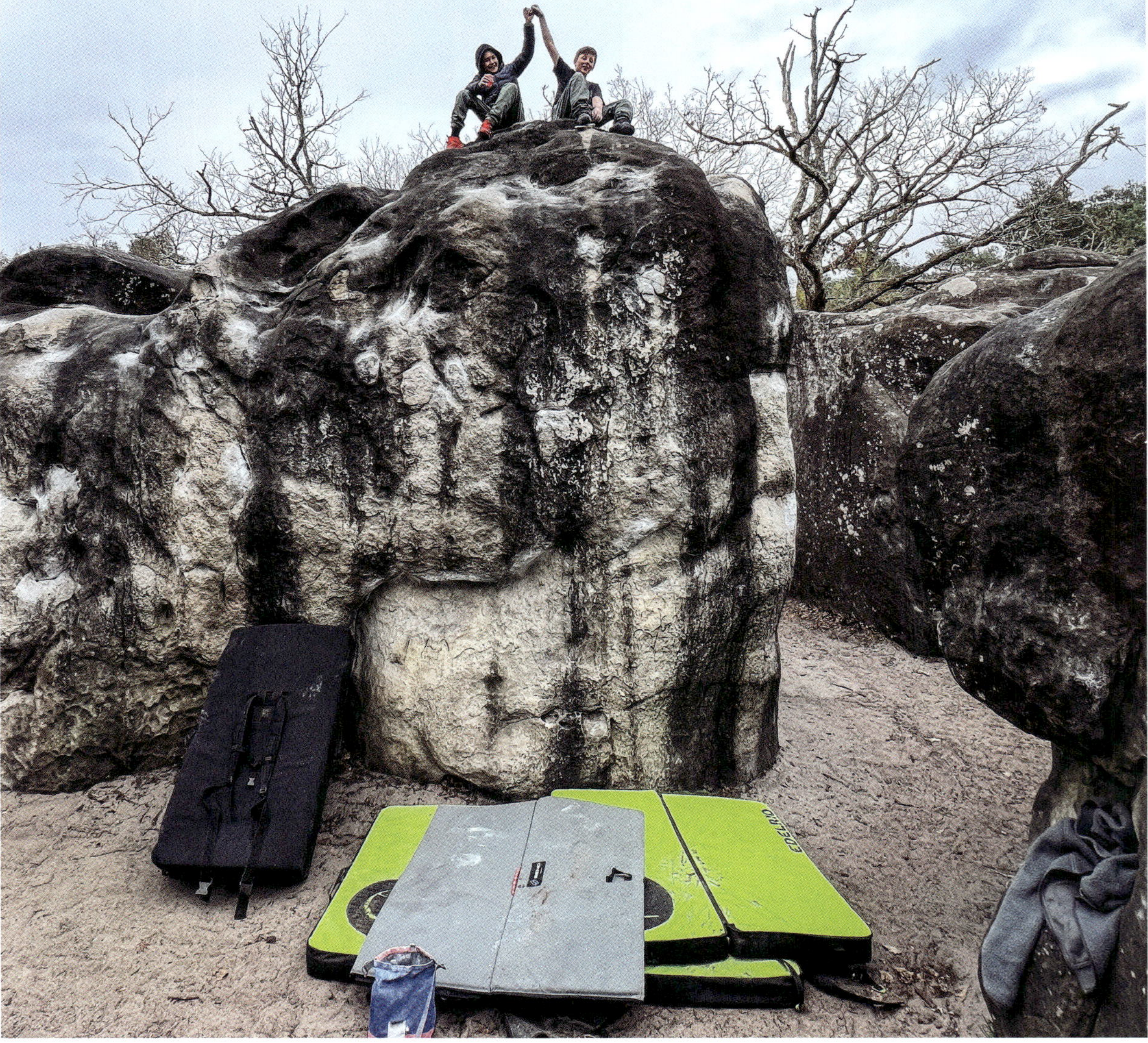

Two happy boys at the top of a boulder in Fontainebleau.

SHOULDERS

After the fingers, the shoulders are the next most common site of injury for climbers. However, unlike in the fingers, there are far more structures in and around the shoulder that are susceptible to injury, and it is beyond the scope of this book to describe all of these in detail. Instead, I will describe the most common climbing-related injuries and look at how we should handle them as effectively as possible.

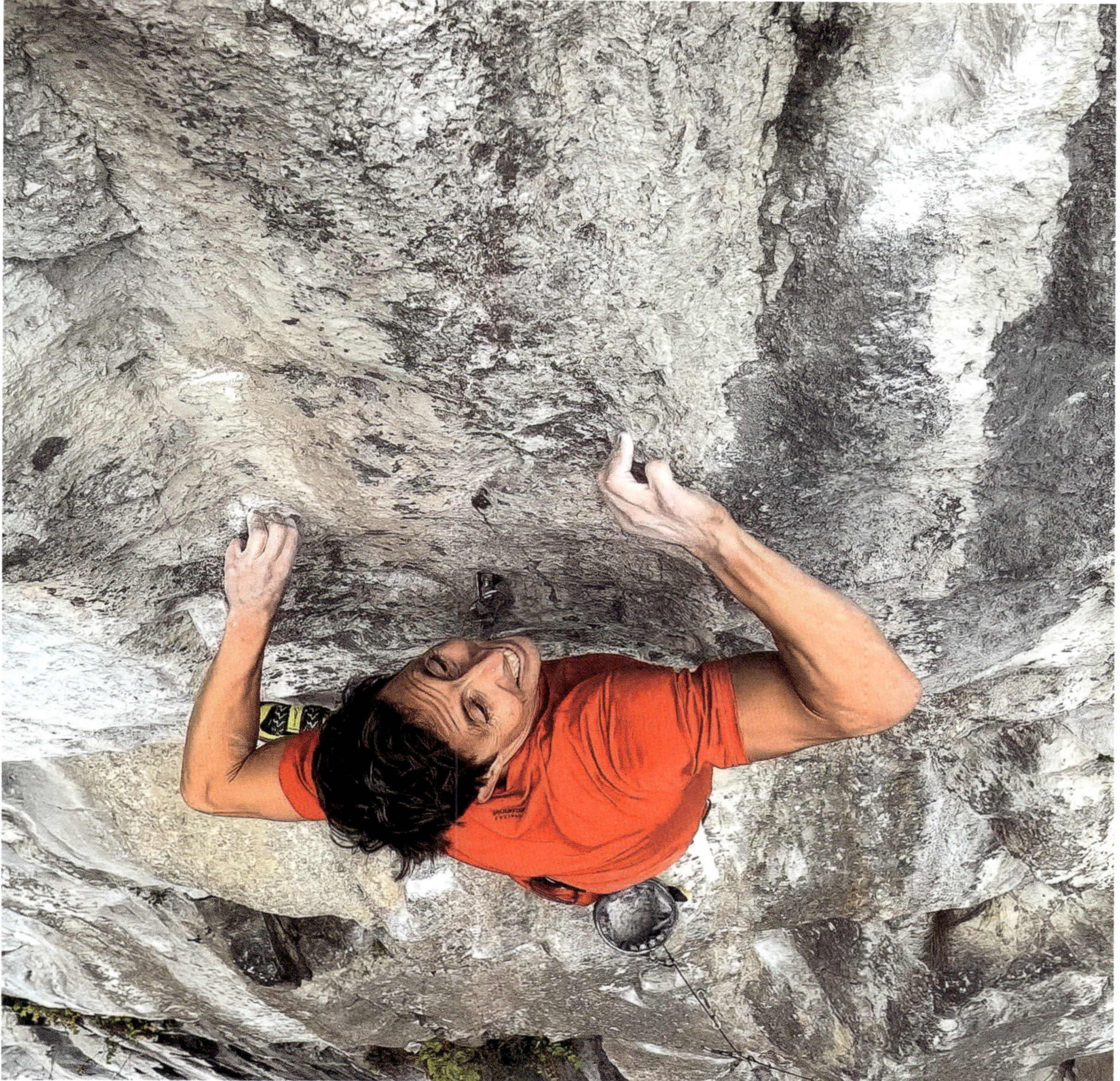

The author in a double shoulder press on the first ascent of *Reisen til Ixtlan* (F9a), Hvarnes, Norway.

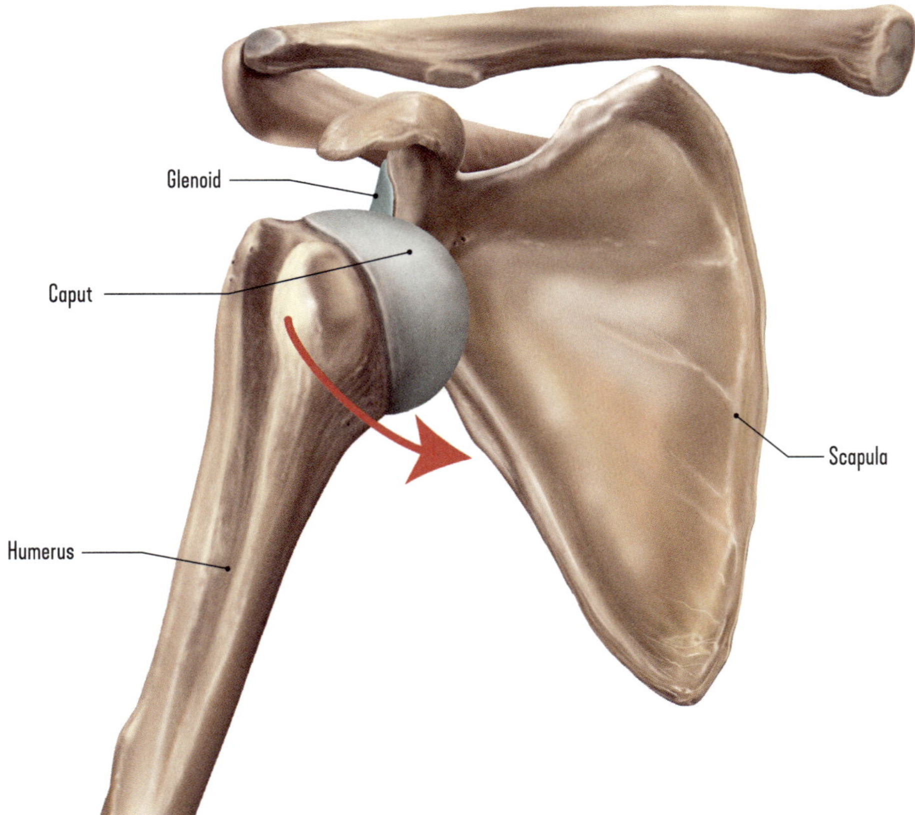

ANTERIOR SHOULDER DISLOCATION

If the shoulder dislocates as a result of an acute event, such as a fall or a heinous move, it will dislocate forwards in over 90 per cent of cases.

This dislocation involves the head of the upper arm bone sliding out of its socket in the shoulder blade. In some cases, it happens as a subluxation (partial dislocation), where immediately after dislocation it slips back into place on its own; however, it will usually remain dislocated and must be put back into place. Once this is done, an X-ray image should be taken to rule out fractures and ensure that the shoulder joint is properly positioned.

Since dislocating the shoulder involves structural damage to the joint, an MRI examination is also recommended to assess the labrum, the joint capsule and the rotator cuff tendons. This is important for assessing the stabilising structures, because the more structural damage there is, the greater the likelihood of future dislocations. And despite a thorough rehabilitation programme, unfortunately the chance of a subsequent dislocation is high, especially in younger and active people. Therefore, the situation should be discussed with an orthopaedic surgeon regarding whether surgical stabilisation should be considered or if the focus should be on rehabilitation and a return to climbing instead.

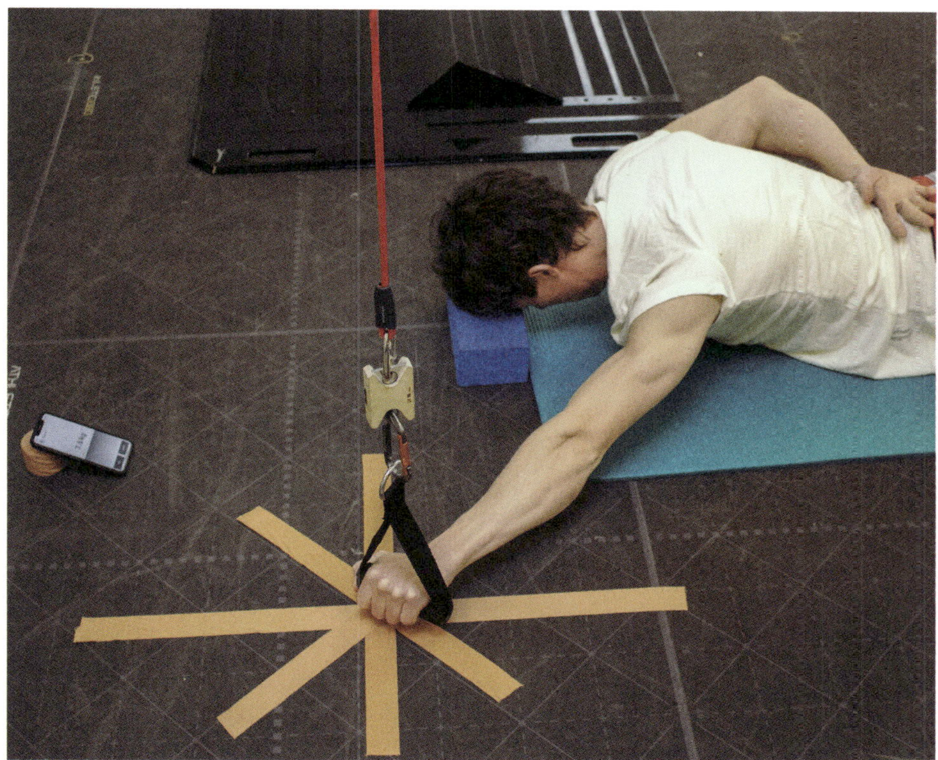

The ASH test is one of many options for the monitoring of shoulder and glenohumeral strength development during rehabilitation following an anterior shoulder dislocation.

Repeated dislocations cause more damage to the stabilising structures in and around the shoulder joint, thus further increasing the risk of recurring dislocations. These are important considerations to take into account when deciding whether or not to consider surgery.

Initially, the pain will limit how much the arm can be used, but it is still appropriate to start training from an early stage to stimulate the muscles without risking another shoulder dislocation.

The exercise selection can be done both with and without occlusion (see box-out), with the goal of preserving muscle mass and creating movement of the shoulder joint. In consultation with healthcare professionals, progression should continue towards heavier loads, increased range of motion and faster movements. The focus must always be on putting yourself in the best possible position to return to climbing, so the training should be both general *and* sport specific.

EARLY PHASE EXERCISES

OCCLUSION TRAINING

This is also known as blood flow resistance training (BFRT), and the principle is to reduce the venous blood flow from the muscles.

Occlusion of blood flow leads to reduced oxygen supply and an accumulation of waste products in the muscles, thus increasing the metabolic stress, which is what we aim for when working a muscle to fatigue.

The combination of mechanical load and metabolic stress results in muscle growth, or at least a reduction of muscle loss during a period when we cannot load the muscles as before. The advantage of using straps to restrict circulation is that we can get away with both lower load and lower volume in an exercise, and yet still stimulate the muscles.

The exercise protocols presented here can be done with 1 set of 30 repetitions followed by 3 sets of 15 repetitions. Start with exercise 1 and work through all exercises before starting the next set. It should be uncomfortable but not painful, and there has been no evidence showing better training effect by increasing pressure.

The goal is to work with a constant pumping sensation without pain or tingling/stinging in the arms.

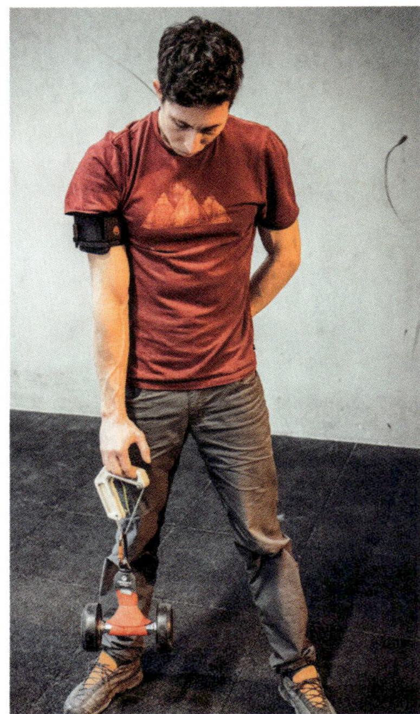

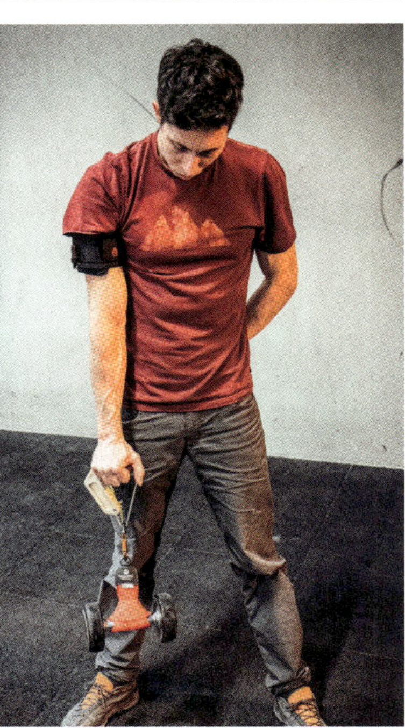

EXERCISE 1: **FINGER CURLS.** Using a light weight or resistance band, curl your fingers from an open position to a closed curl.

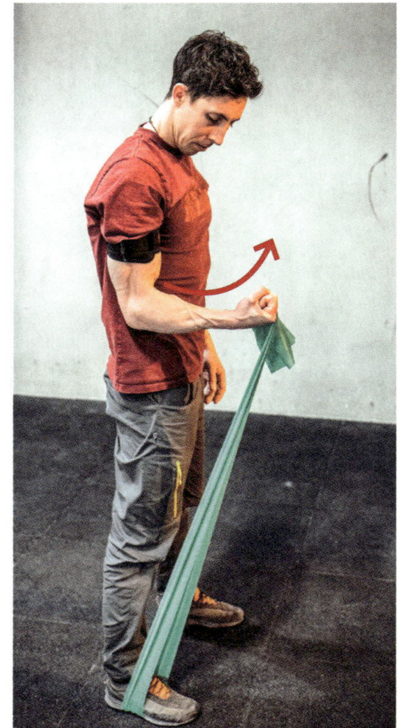

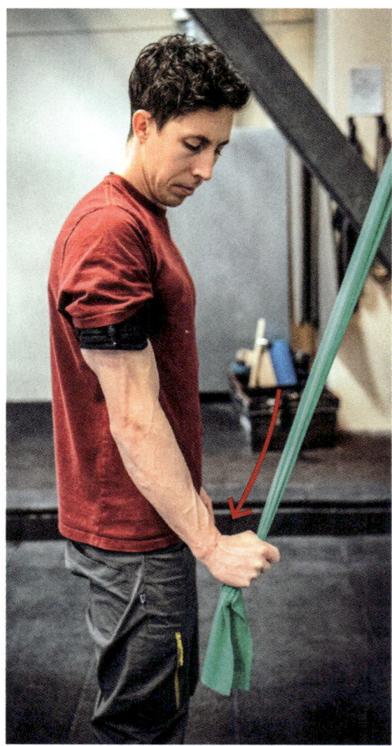

EXERCISES 2 AND 3: **BICEPS CURLS** and **TRICEPS PRESS.**

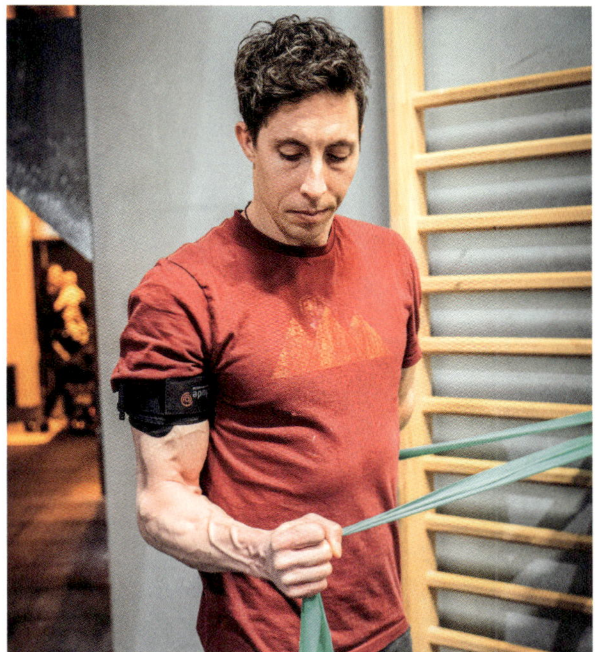

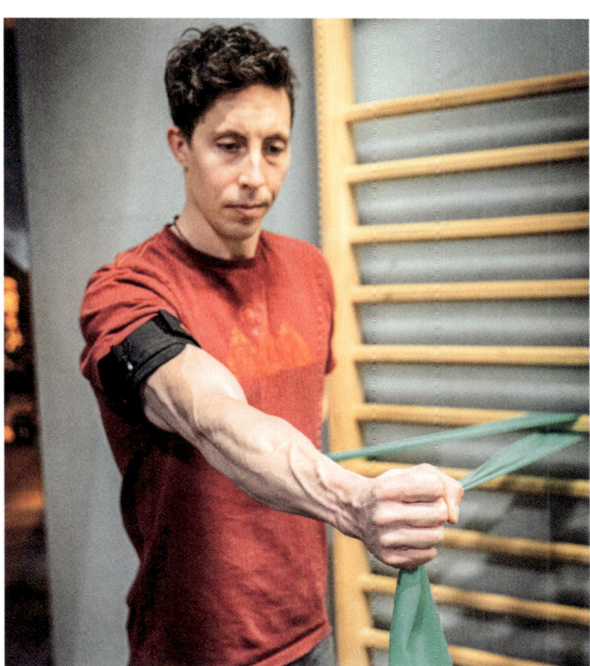

EXERCISE 4: PALLOF PRESS. Start with your arm at your side and your elbow at a 90-degree angle. Press your arm straight forwards without it moving in front of your body.

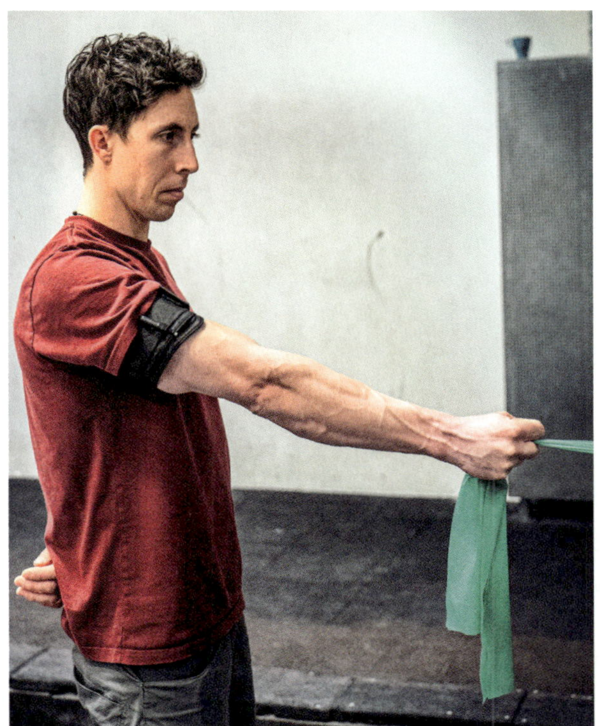

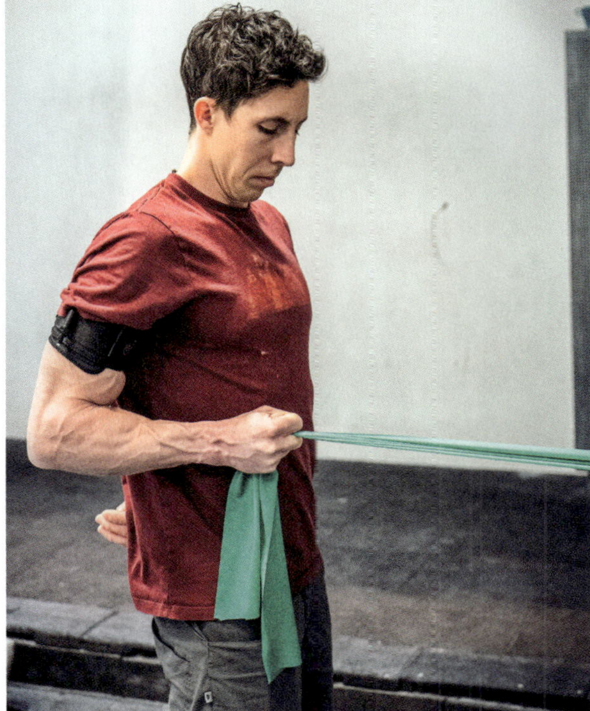

EXERCISE 5: ROWING. Starting with a straight arm, pull straight backwards, at the same time pulling your shoulder blade back and towards the centre.

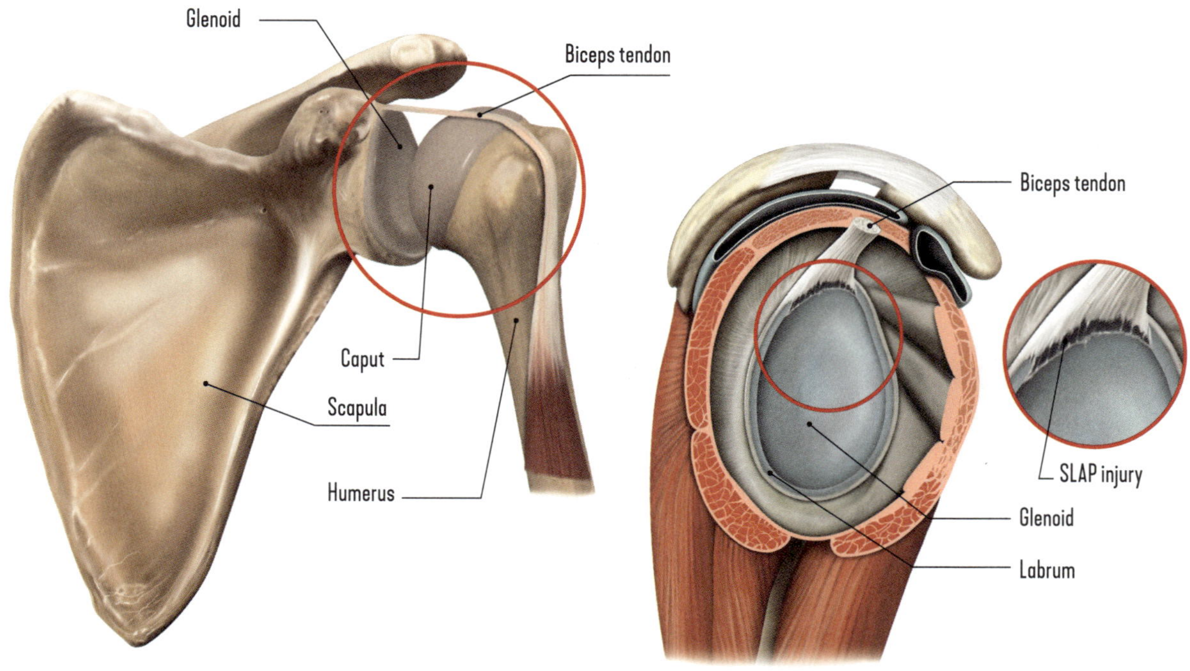

BICEPS AND LABRUM

Around the glenoid cavity of the scapula, we have a labrum that functions as a suction cup on the joint head. This labrum allows the joint head to move around in the glenoid cavity without dislocating. At the upper aspect of this labrum, the tendon from the long head of the biceps attaches, and this site of the labrum can be damaged due to both acute trauma and microtraumas over time. When this injury is seen on MRI images, it is called SLAP – *superior labral anterior to posterior* – where the acronym describes an injury to the upper labrum that extends from the anterior (front) part to the posterior (back) part of the glenoid.

The mechanism of injury involves stress that causes the biceps tendon to pull the labrum off the bone, which can result in pain, clicking in the joint and a feeling of instability. However, such injuries, and changes in the biceps-labrum complex, are regularly observed on MRI images of athletes without any shoulder symptoms, so medical history becomes crucial for further management.

If you have had an acute incident and felt something happen inside your shoulder – for example, while taking a swing on a straight arm, or during a heinous shoulder press – and then experienced subsequent pain and a sense of instability, followed by an MRI showing a SLAP tear, these findings can be correlated. Since the labrum will not reattach itself to the glenoid, surgical stabilisation may be considered if systematic rehabilitation does not fully resolve the condition. Without a triggering traumatic event, there is much uncertainty about whether surgery would be beneficial; however, an individualised and well-designed strength and conditioning programme can allow most climbers to return to their desired level without undergoing surgery to the biceps-labrum complex.

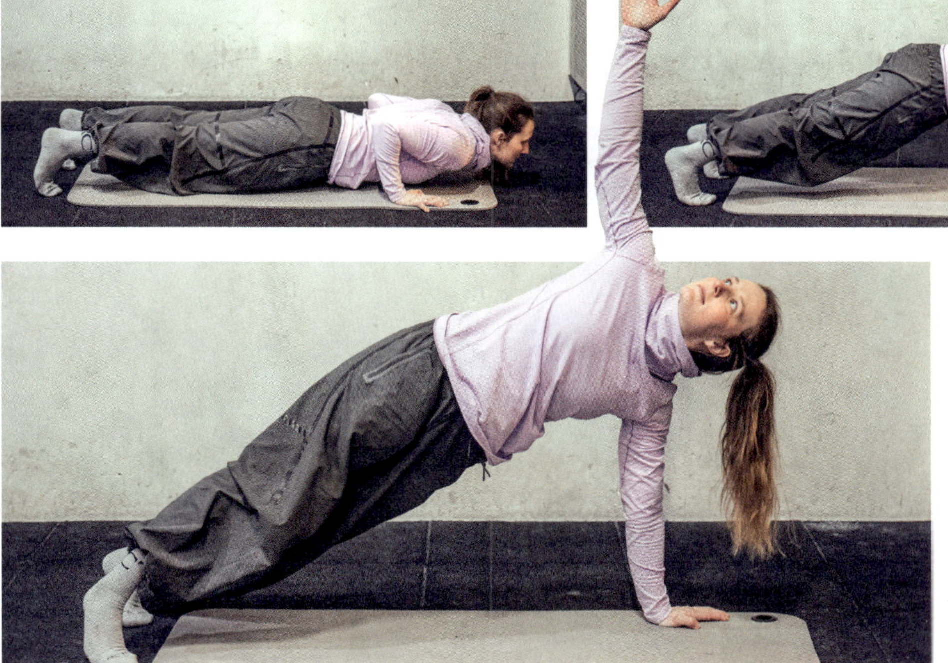

PUSH-UP WITH ROTATION. Do a push-up, then put all your weight on one arm and rotate your torso so that your free arm is pointing up towards the ceiling; repeat with the other side. Do 6–10 repetitions and 3 sets.

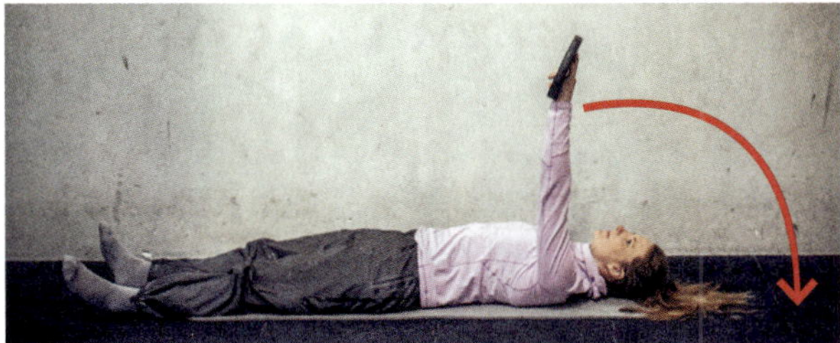

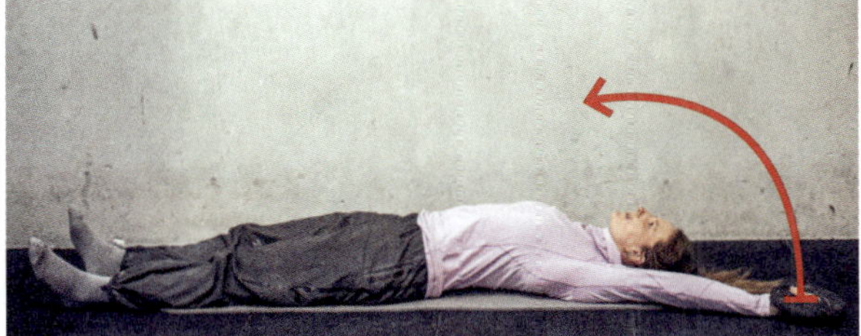

PULL-OVER. Lie on your back and hold a weight disc in one hand. Bring your arm straight back and down towards the floor. Make sure to keep your back in contact with the floor so that it doesn't arch upwards to help you lower your arm. Note that the bottom position is the most demanding, so adjust the weight so that you have control in this part of the movement. Do 6–8 repetitions and 3 sets as part of your warm-up for climbing, or as part of a strength training programme.

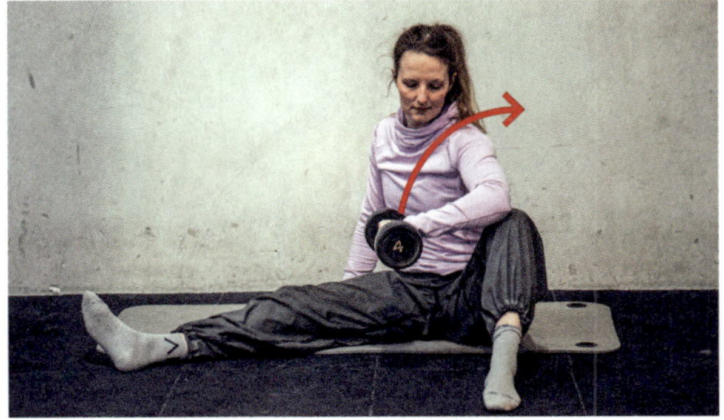

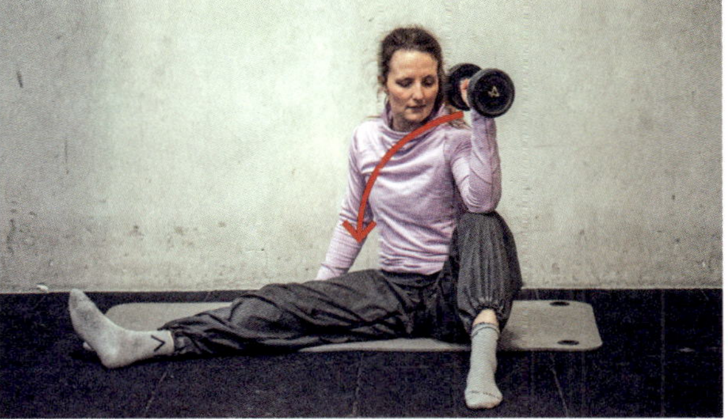

SUPPORTED EXTERNAL ROTATION. Holding a dumb-bell, let your arm rest on the inside of your knee with a 90-degree angle in the elbow joint. Bring your arm up so that the weight is pointing towards the ceiling and then slowly lower it back down. Repeat for 6–8 repetitions and 3 sets.

EXERCISES

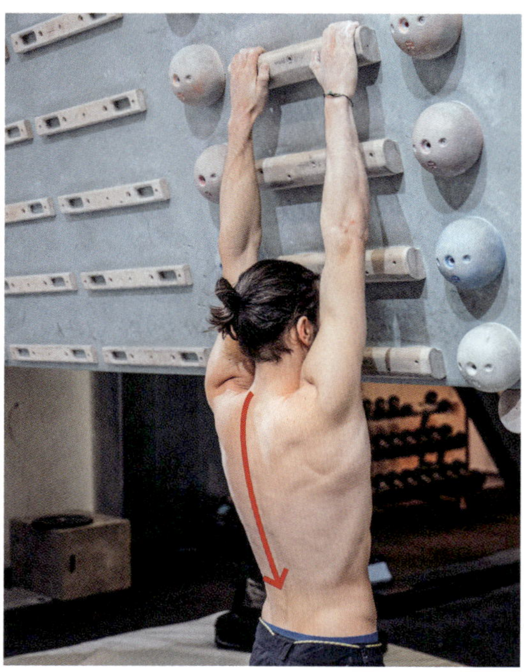

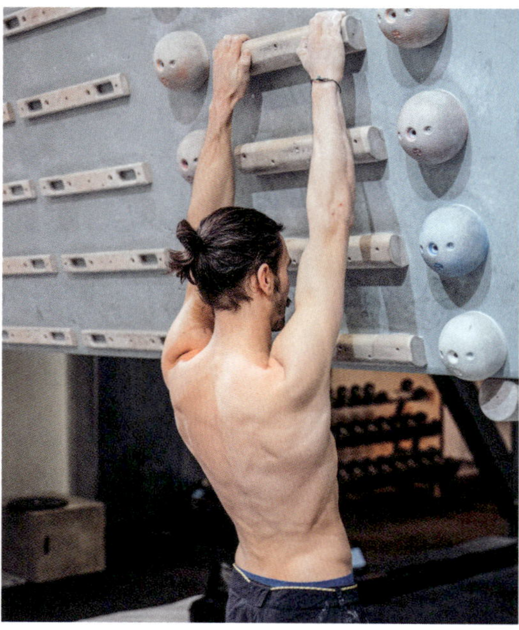

SCAPULAR PULL-UP. Hang on straight arms and pull your shoulder blades down and back so that you end up in a higher position but with your arms still straight. Slowly lower back down and repeat for 6–10 repetitions in 2 sets as part of your climbing warm-up (see page 34).

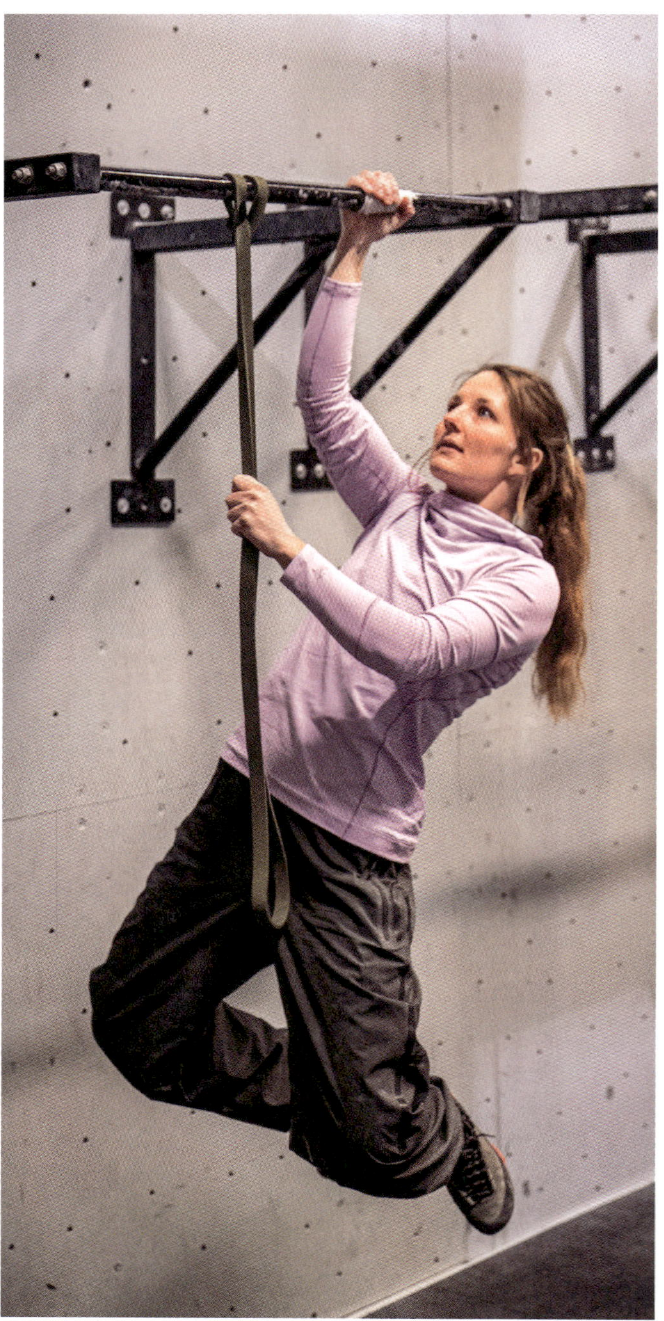

ONE-ARM LOCK-OFF IN OPEN POSITION. With an open position (wider than 90 degrees of elbow flexion), the upper arm is farther away from the body than when locking off in a higher position, placing greater demands on the adduction muscles around the shoulder joint. Hold this position for 10 seconds until you are close to exhaustion at the end of the hang; repeat for 3 sets. I recommend gradually reducing the hang time to 3–5 seconds and increasing the weight.

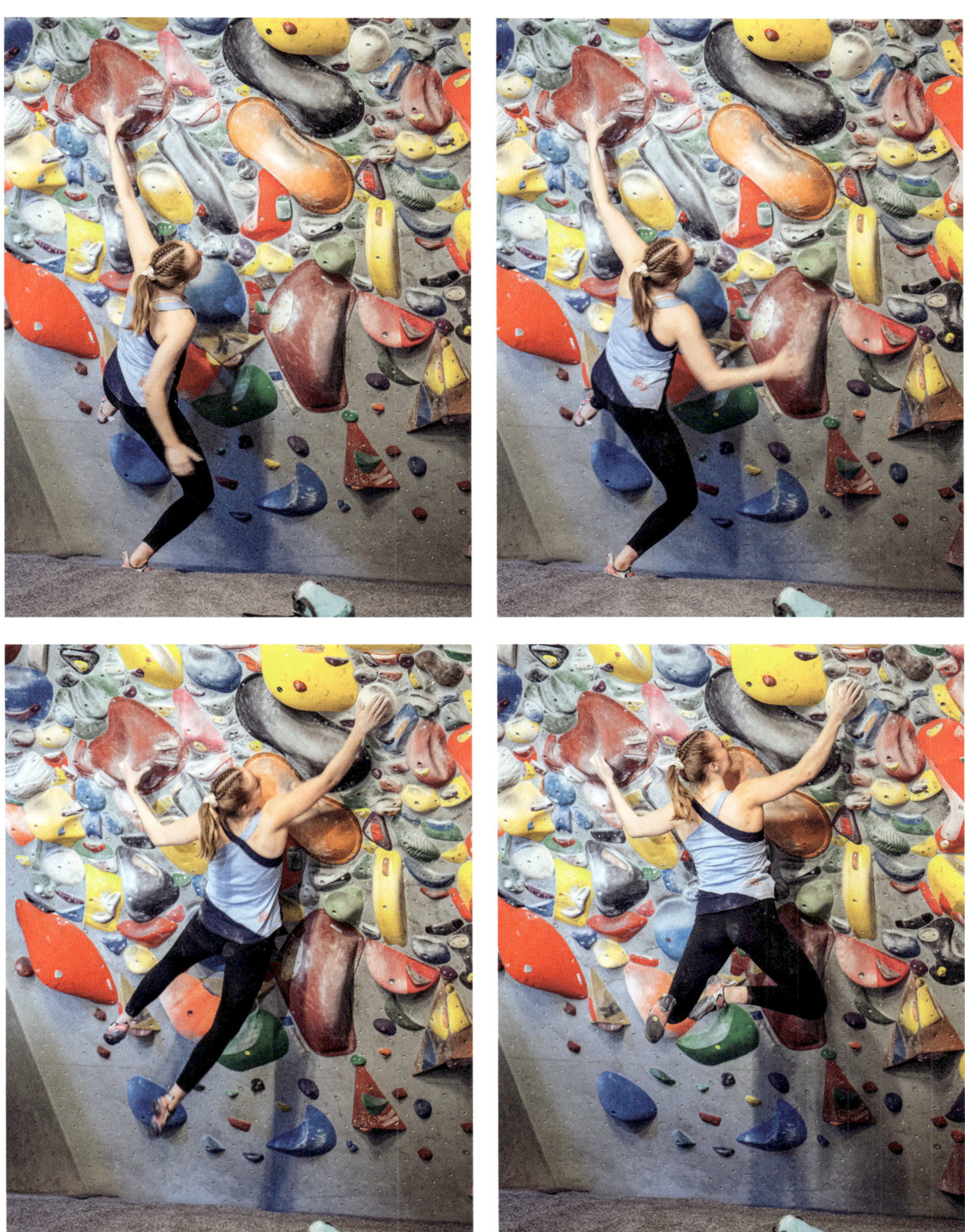

JUMP-START. On a spray wall, you can practise jump-starts with different holds and varying distances between them. Large distances between holds require more strength and stability, so start with a short distance and increase the distance as you get stronger and more confident.

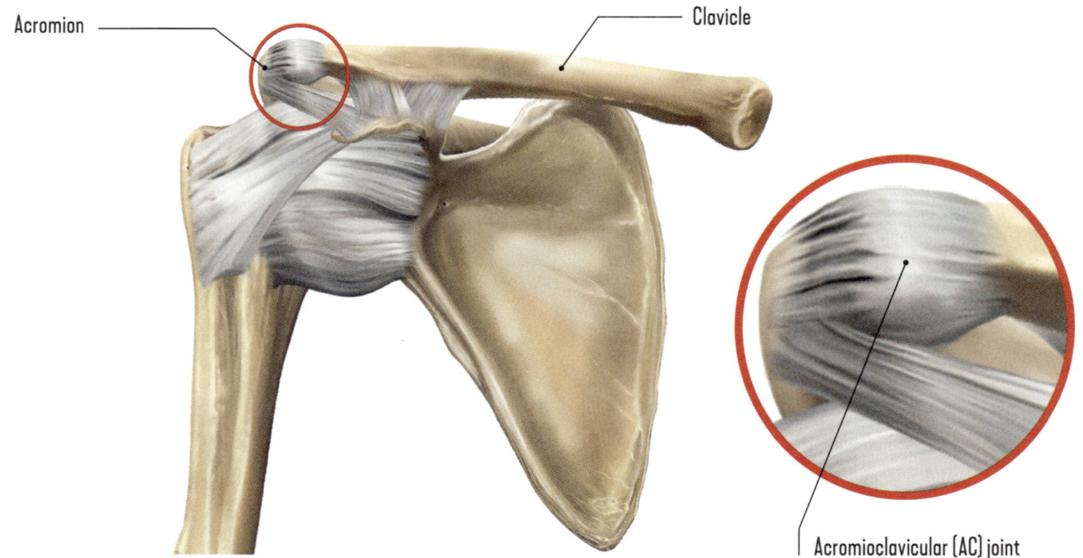

AC JOINT

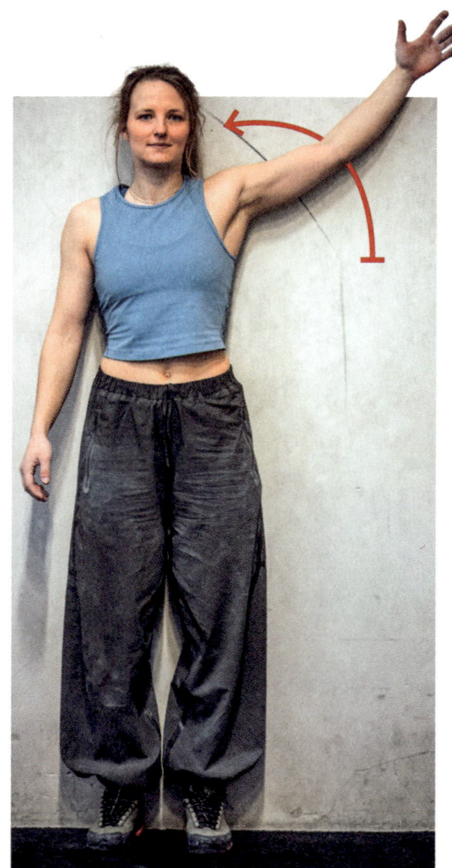

If the pain above the AC joint increases the higher you lift your arm, it is called 'high-arc pain'. This is a characteristic of AC joint-related pain.

The joint between the shoulder blade and collarbone is called the acromioclavicular joint, also known as the AC joint. The AC joint can be dislocated in a fall, and these injuries must be examined to determine their severity. The majority of such injuries are treated without surgery, and rehabilitation is guided by pain and range of motion; the prognosis is good.

For climbers, load-related AC joint pain is more common than fall-related pain. It can occur spontaneously, for example following a demanding shoulder move, or over time as a result of hanging from straight arms. The pain is localised at the top of the shoulder and is caused by irritation or inflammation within the joint. Like with the finger joints, excessive load affects the AC joint when the articular surfaces are compressed against one other. The key to resolving the problem is managing load and avoiding positions known to compress the joint, such as when the arm is fully elevated overhead or when the upper arm crosses the midline, such as during a shoulder press. As long as you're aware of these positions, you can train and climb around them. Symptoms often worsen if you try to work through these positions despite experiencing pain, but they will typically disappear on their own when you work around them.

More pronounced changes in the joint – i.e. osteoarthritis – may predispose individuals to recurring problems within their AC joints. However, many people diagnosed with arthritis based on X-rays or MRIs do not experience any symptoms from their joints; therefore, any imaging findings must be considered alongside a clinical examination and whether pain is present or not. For cases involving AC joint arthritis with recurrent inflammation and pain, measures such as cortisone injections and eventually surgery should be discussed with healthcare professionals.

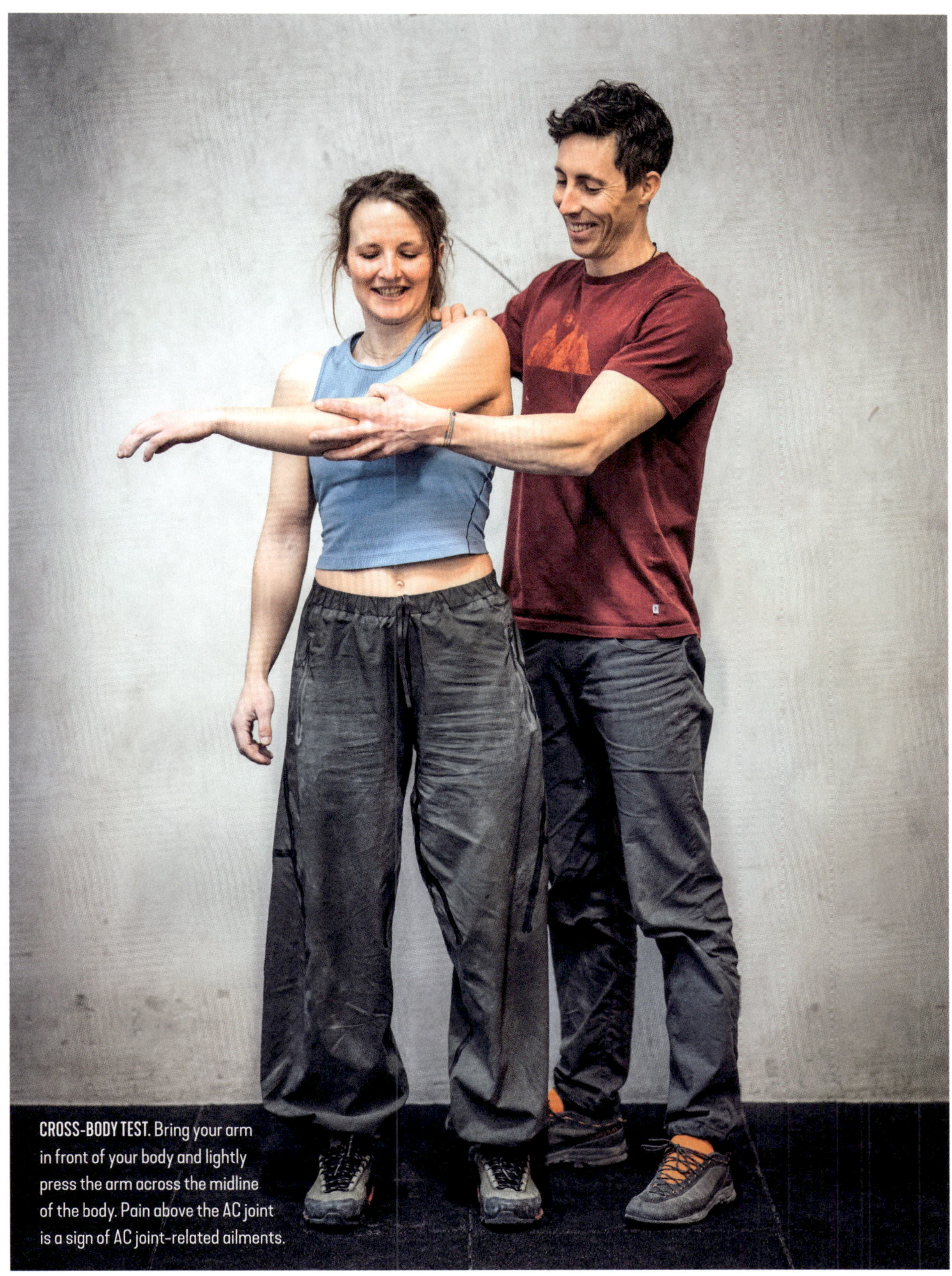

CROSS-BODY TEST. Bring your arm in front of your body and lightly press the arm across the midline of the body. Pain above the AC joint is a sign of AC joint-related ailments.

EXERCISES IN PROGRESSIVE ORDER

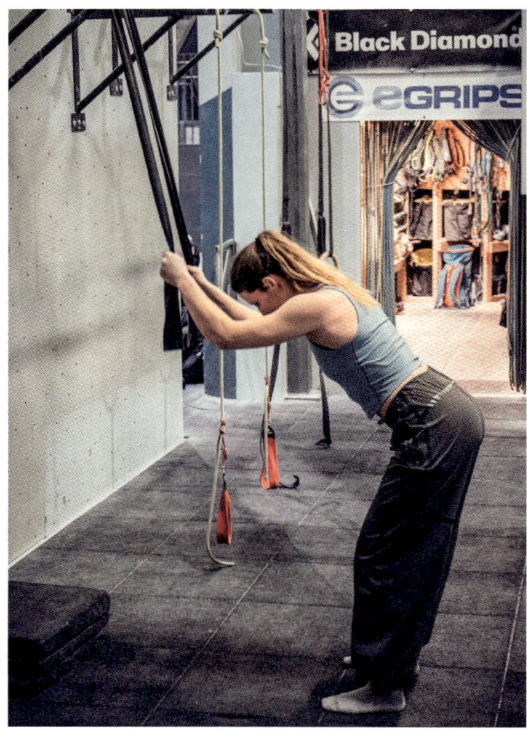

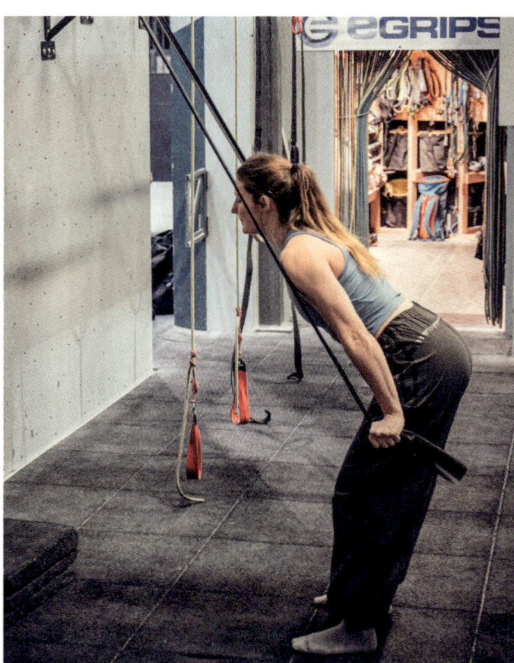

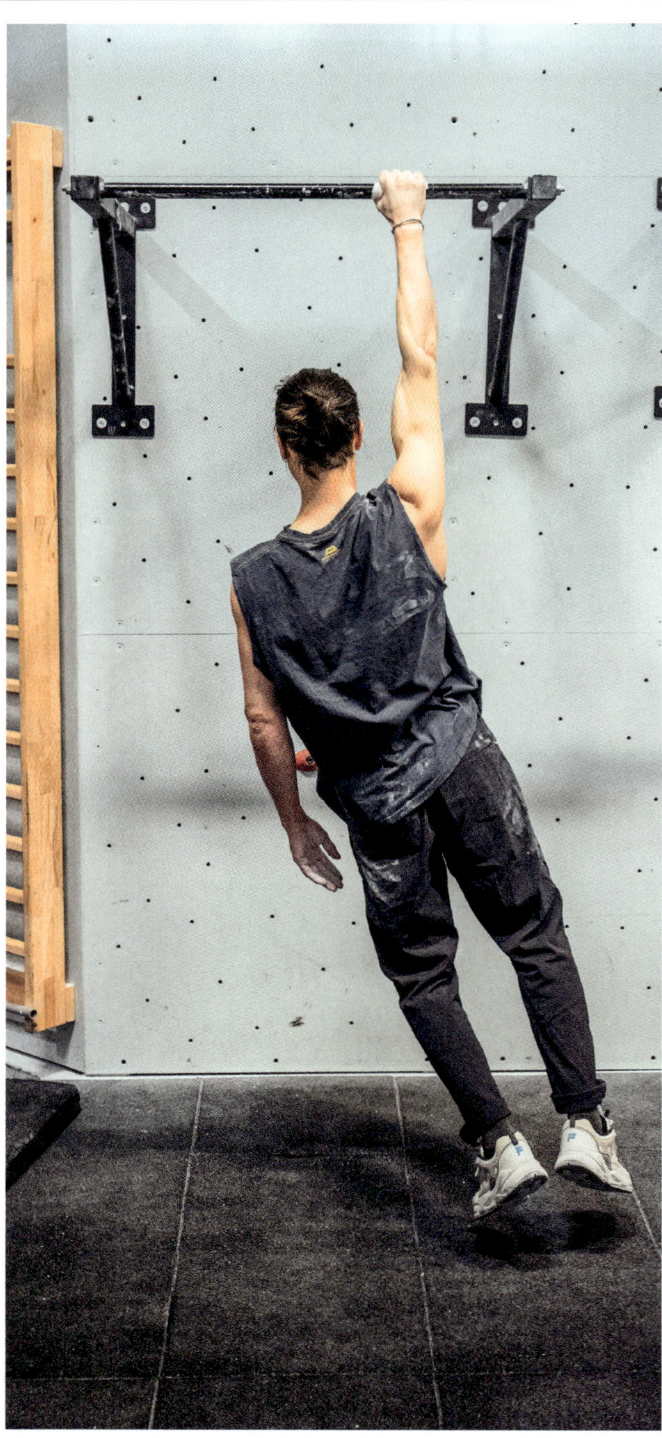

PULL-DOWNS WITH RESISTANCE BAND. Start with your arms at a height that does not provoke symptoms and pull the band down to your hips. This can be done as a warm-up exercise with about 20 repetitions and 2 sets.

ONE-ARM ACTIVE HANG. Find the top position in a scapular pull-up and then hang by only one arm. This can be done with a band for your foot to relieve some weight if it is too heavy with your full body weight. Hold for 5 seconds and repeat for 5 hangs with 30 seconds' rest between hangs.

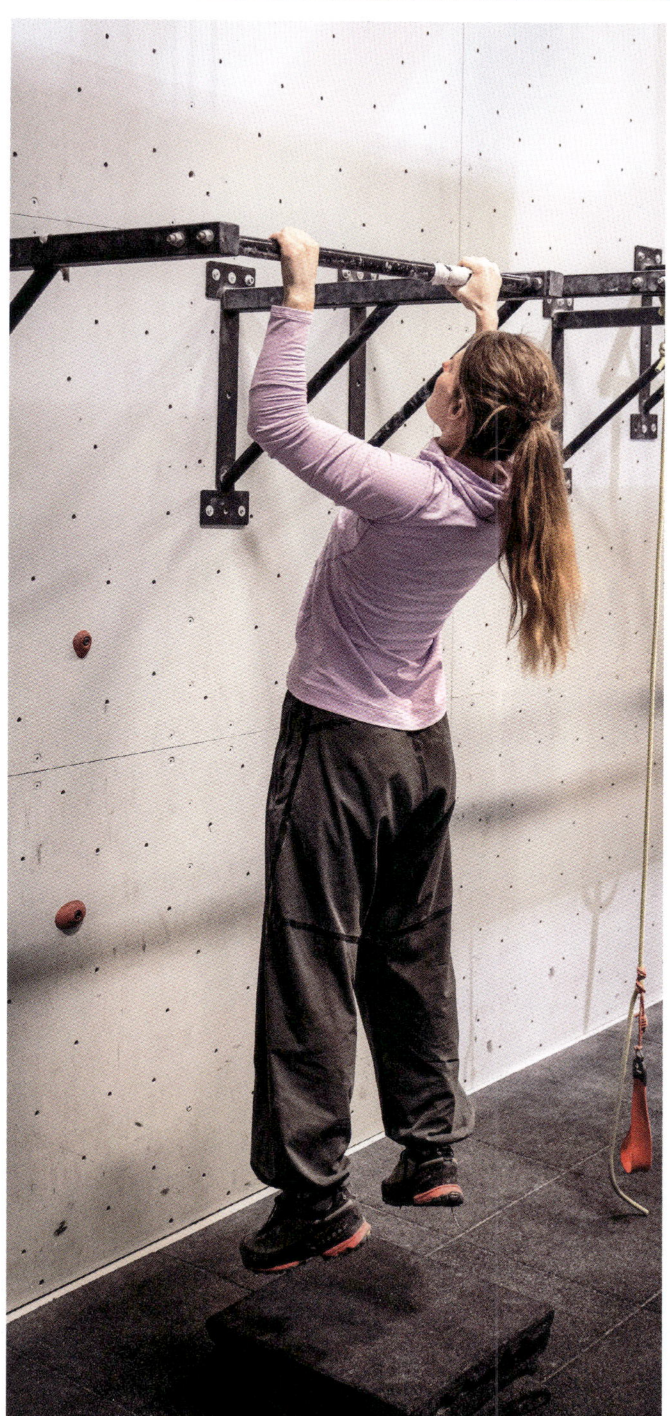

MID-RANGE PULL-UP. It's usually the bottom position, and in some cases the top position, that is troublesome. So, the solution for training strength can be to train in the so-called 'mid-range', i.e. avoiding the outer positions, but training heavily in the part of the movement path that is symptom-free.

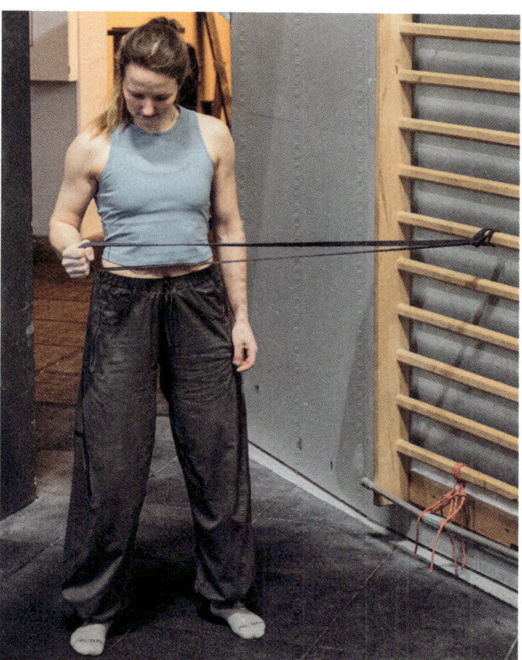

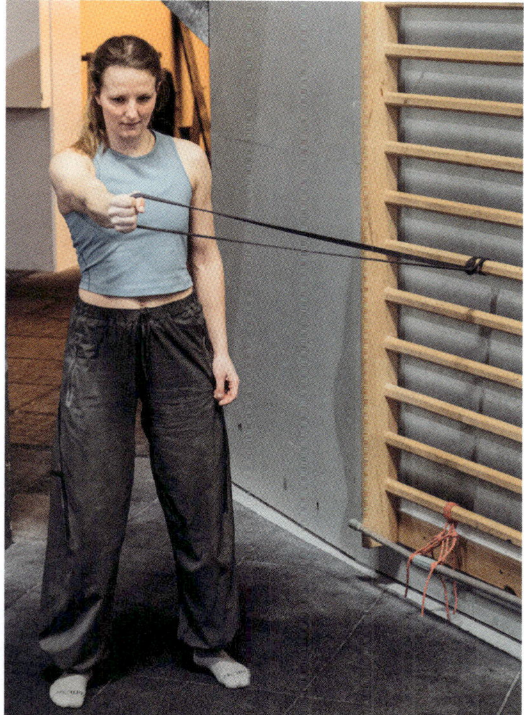

PALLOF PRESS. Start with your arm at your side and your elbow at a 90-degree angle. Press your arm straight forwards, without allowing it to move in front of your body. Do 6–8 repetitions and 3 sets.

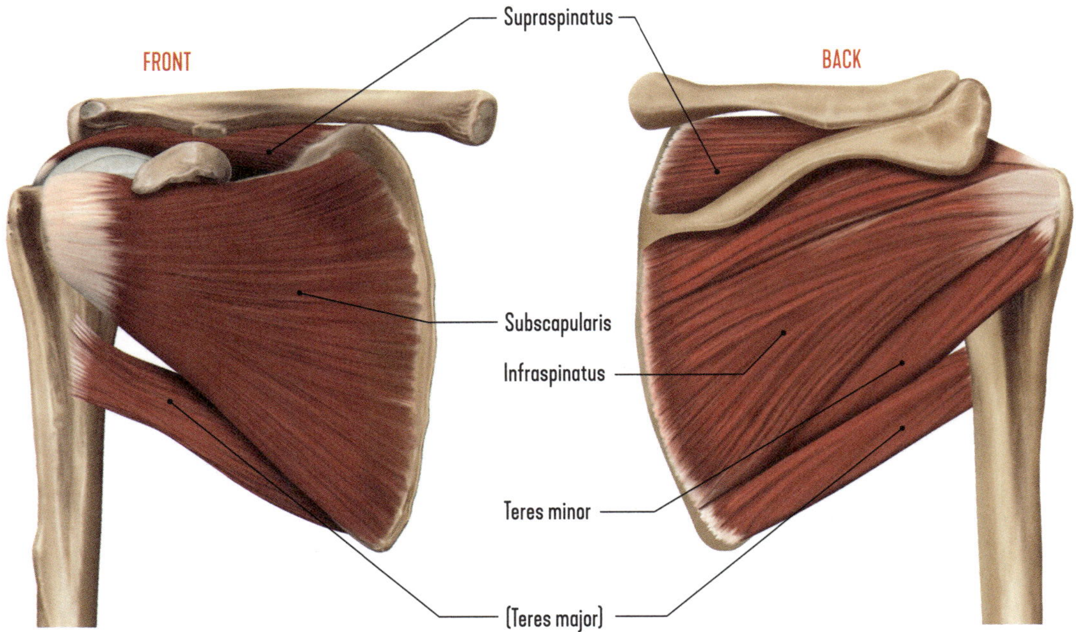

THE ROTATOR CUFF

The rotator cuff is a collection of four muscles – supraspinatus, subscapularis, infraspinatus and teres minor – with their associated tendons that attach as a cuff around the head of the upper arm. The shoulder joint can be compared to a ball (the head) resting in a socket (the glenoid), and it is this relationship between the ball and the socket that makes the shoulder the most mobile joint in the body. However, mobility comes at the expense of stability, and the main job of the rotator cuff is to centre the ball in the socket when we move the arm.

As a result of traumas such as falls or other acute incidents, the rotator cuff tendons can rupture, and large cuff tears involving multiple tendons should be treated by an orthopaedic surgeon. The clinical signs of such injuries are an acute event followed by loss of strength and function of the arm. This strength loss is called a *lag sign*, and includes difficulties lifting the arm sideways, rotating the arm outwards or putting the arm behind the back. While pain may make it difficult to develop strength, lag signs are indicative of a tendon rupture where the muscle is no longer attached to the bone; reduced strength due to pain is another phenomenon, one that is also much more common than loss of strength due to extensive tendon tears.

Minor and partial tears of one or more rotator cuff tendons are relatively common. Like larger tears, smaller ones can occur acutely, but, generally, when examining people without shoulder pain or any previous shoulder injury, small tears are not uncommon in people aged 30 and older. Changes in tendon tissue are thus understood as processes that occur over time, and, similar to the elbow tendinopathies described earlier (pages 86–95), they do not necessarily cause pain. Therefore, these small, partial rotator cuff tendon ruptures

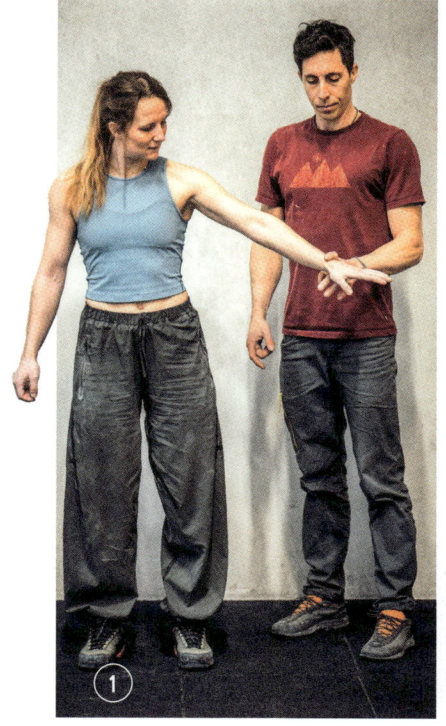

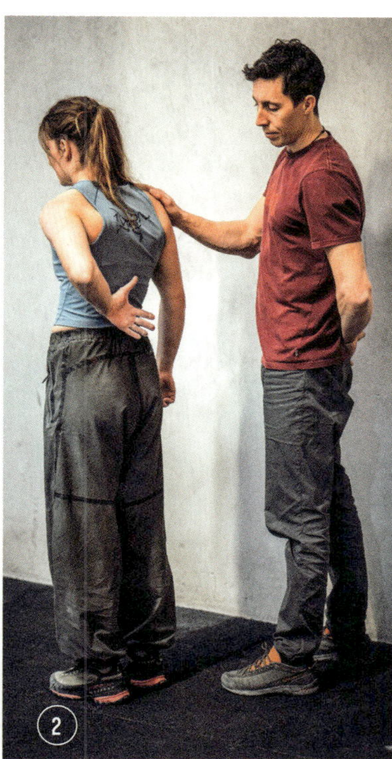

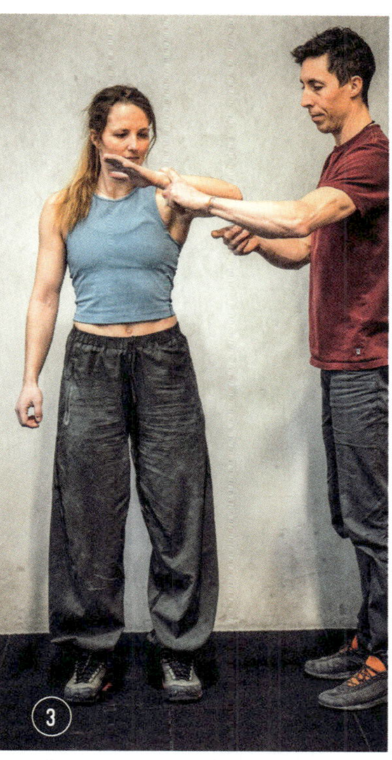

LAG SIGN is the inability to perform a movement or maintain a position. Here we test abduction (photo 1), internal rotation (photo 2) and external rotation (photo 3 (Hornblower)). The inability to perform the movement, or the fact that it only takes the force of one finger to break the position, indicates greater damage to the rotator cuff. Consequently, you should be referred for further investigation.

fall under the tendinopathy concept (pages 92–93) when they are considered as the cause of symptoms – and they are managed accordingly.

The term *rotator cuff tendinopathy* is therefore proposed as a way to understand non-traumatic shoulder problems, and when these small tears are seen as part of the tendinopathy it means that tendon-related issues can occur even without ruptures. A symptom of tendon-related problems is pain on loading. The strength is there, but it hurts to use the arm. Through a review of someone's medical history and a clinical examination, we can identify probable triggers – which positions and movements increase symptoms – and then develop a plan for how to best manage the condition.

It might come as a surprise to learn that this plan will not include the classic rotational exercises with bands that have been recommended for years. The rotator cuff has multiple jobs, but, as noted earlier, its main job is to stabilise the ball in the socket when we move the arm. So, in order to train the rotator cuff effectively, we must therefore expose it to demands that increase its capacity to tolerate the load, movements and arm positions it will be exposed to when we go climbing. A combination of varied and sport-specific strength training is thus considered the most appropriate approach, and if we can manage this while simultaneously addressing the triggers, most people will experience relief from their symptoms and be able to return to their desired climbing level.

EXERCISES

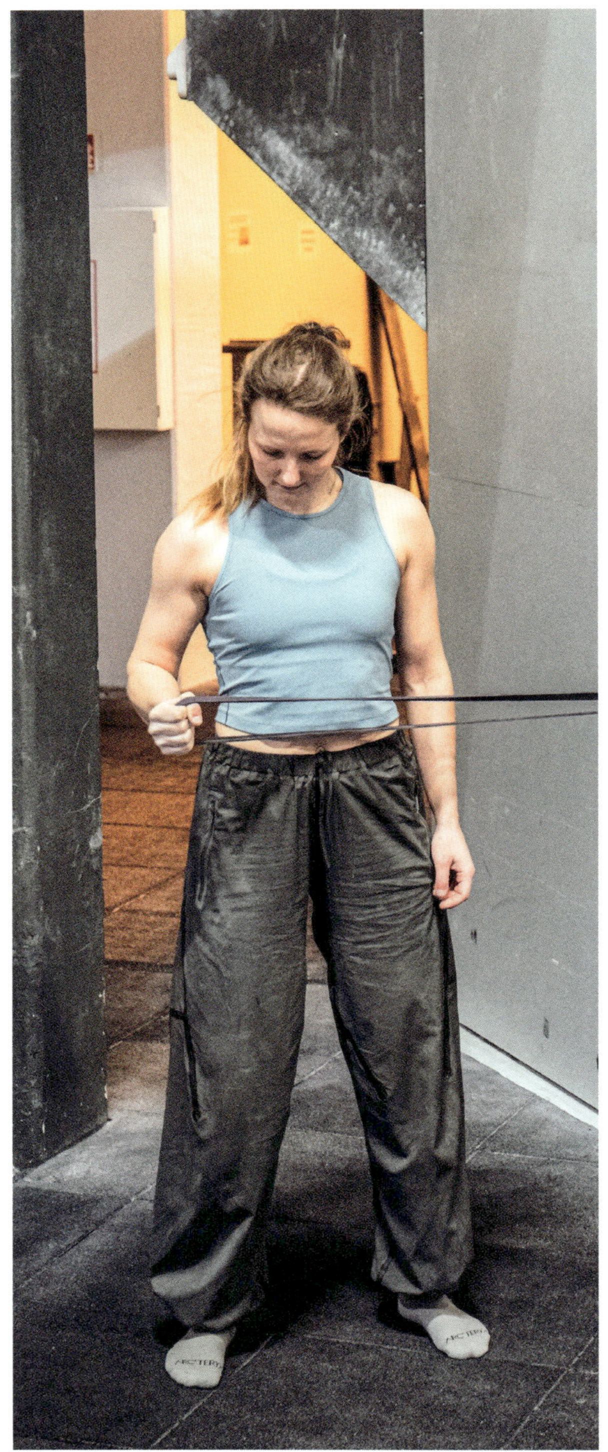

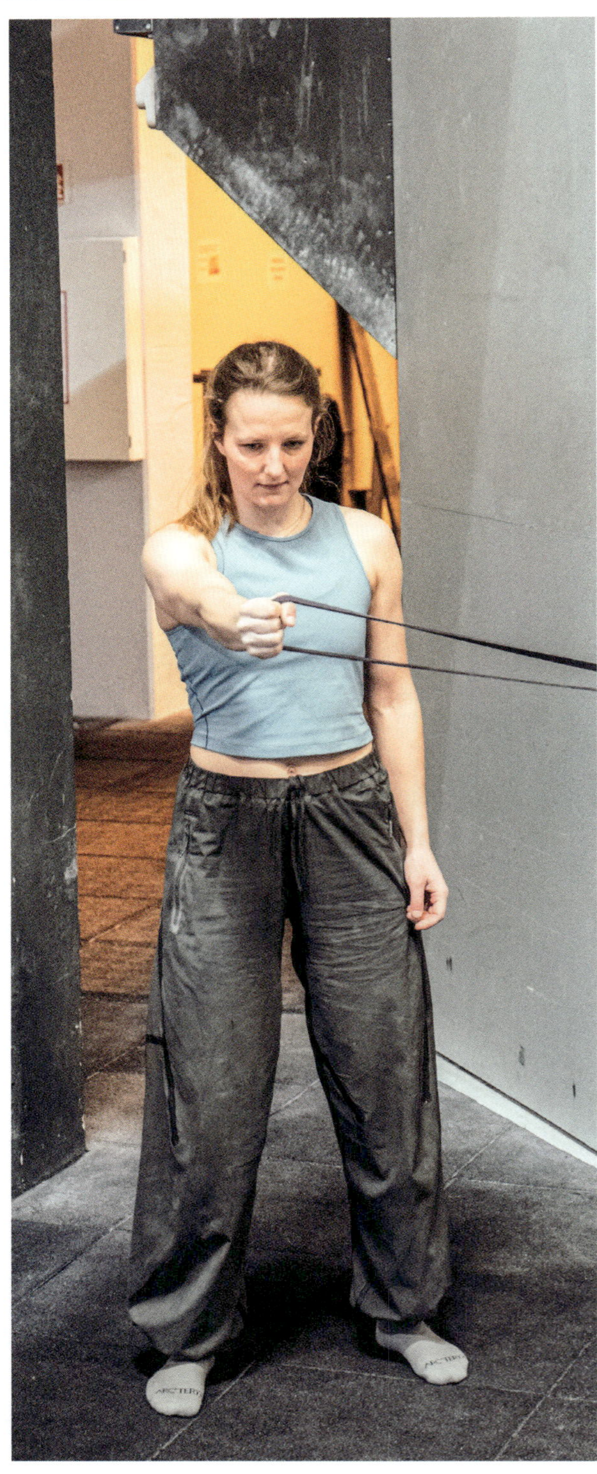

PALLOF PRESS. Start with your arm at your side and your elbow at a 90-degree angle. Push your arm straight forwards without allowing it to move in front of your body. This will work the upper and rear parts of the rotator cuff (supraspinatus and infraspinatus). Do 6–8 repetitions and 3 sets.

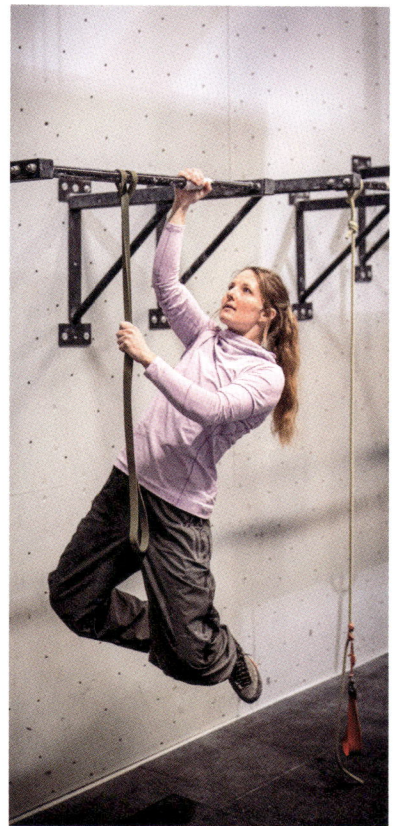

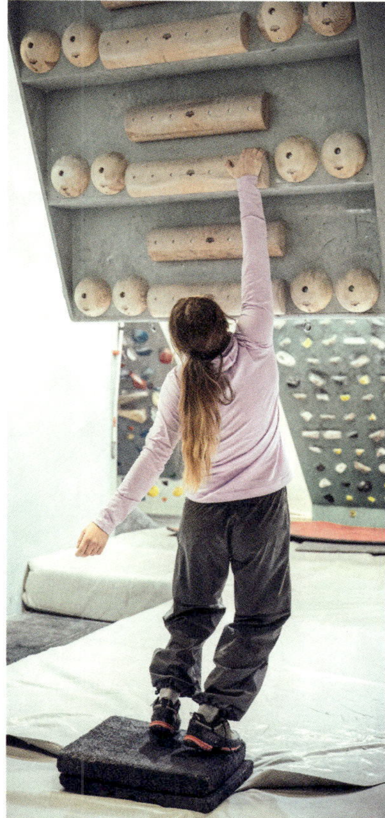

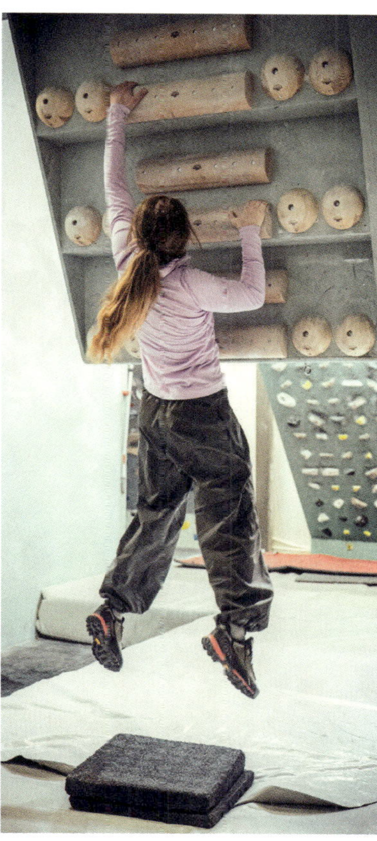

PULLING EXERCISES such as **LOCK-OFF** and **JUMP-START** train the entire shoulder complex, and particularly the front of the rotator cuff (subscapularis). They are climbing-specific and you can train with a high rate of force development, which is an important component in the final part of rehab before returning to sport.

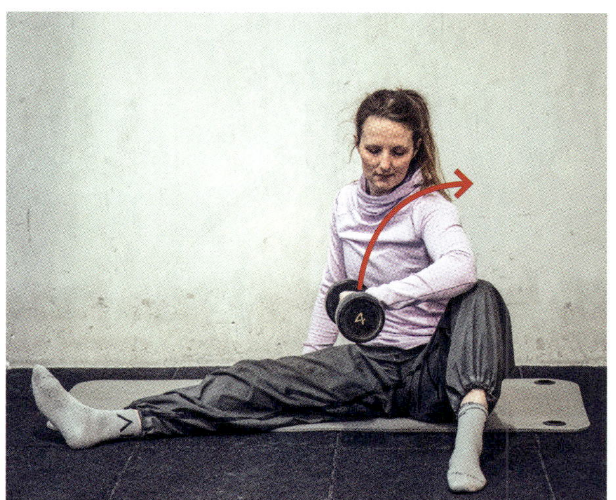

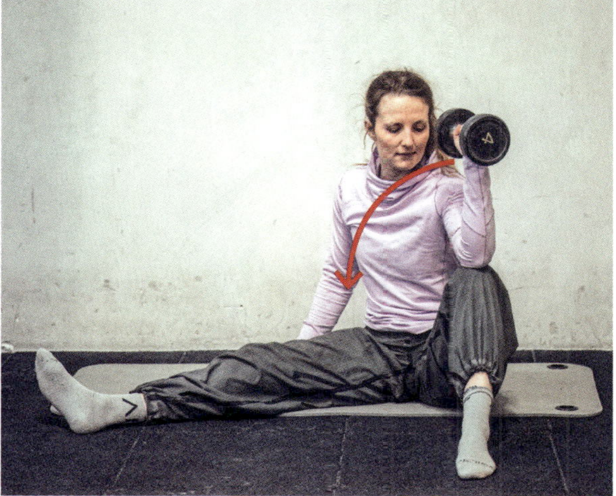

ASSISTED EXTERNAL ROTATION. Holding a dumb-bell, let your arm rest on the inside of your knee with a 90-degree angle at the elbow. Raise your arm so that the weight is pointing towards the ceiling and then slowly lower it back down. Do 6–8 repetitions and 3 sets. This will work the upper and rear parts of the rotator cuff (supraspinatus and infraspinatus).

EXERCISES

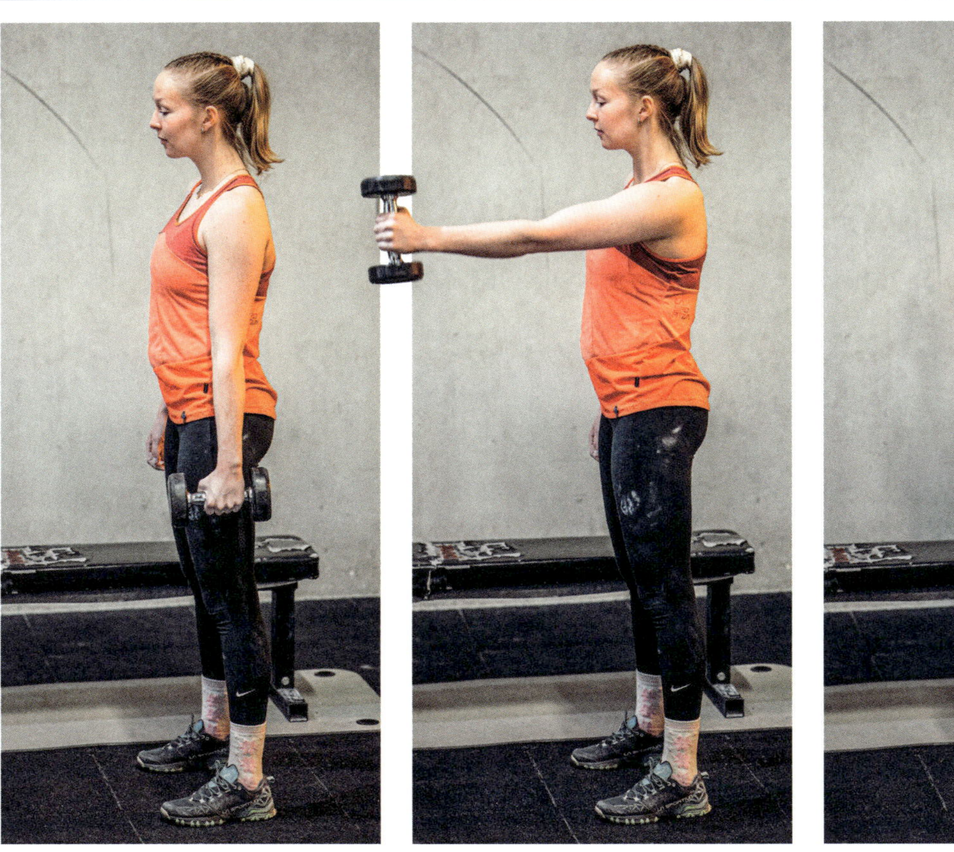

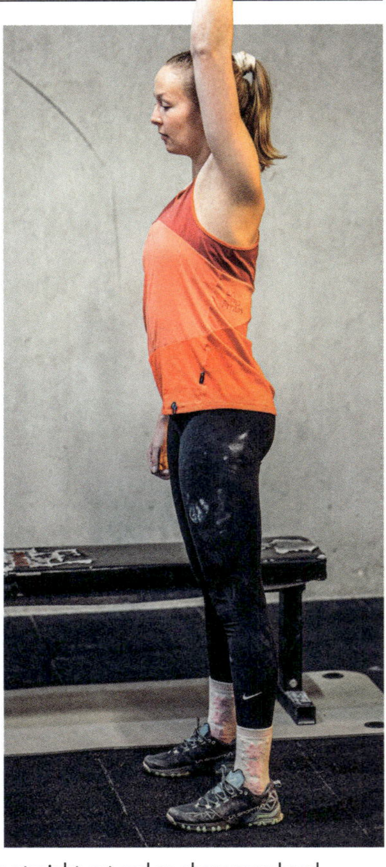

FLEXION RAISE. Starting with your arm by your side and keeping your elbow straight, raise your arm straight out and up above your head. Perform 8–10 repetitions and 2–3 sets. This will work the upper and rear parts of the rotator cuff (supraspinatus and infraspinatus).

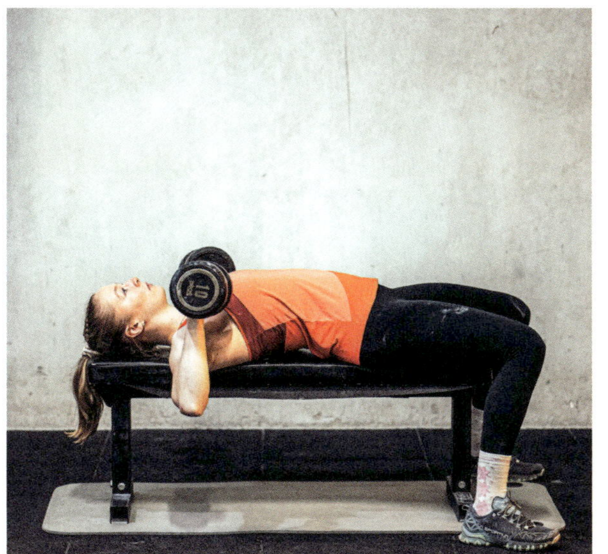

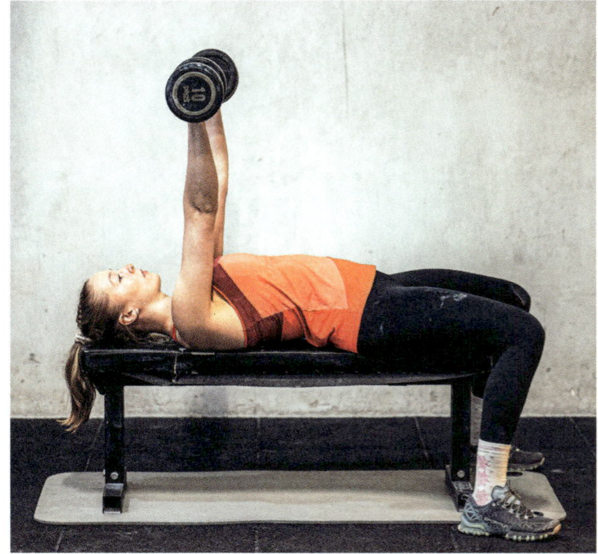

BENCH PRESS WITH DUMB-BELLS. Lie on your back and push the weights straight up towards the ceiling. Slowly lower back down and do 6–8 repetitions and 3 sets to work the upper and rear parts of the rotator cuff (supraspinatus and infraspinatus).

A SHORT AND NERDY SHOULDER STORY

In 1972, orthopaedic surgeon Charles S. Neer introduced the term 'impingement' in reference to shoulder pain. Neer posited that the cause of shoulder pain was the 'pinching' of the rotator cuff tendons and the subacromial bursa underneath the acromion when the arm was raised. This hypothesis was tested by surgically removing the bursa and shaving off the underside of the acromion to increase the subacromial space. As almost all patients became symptom free after this intervention, 'subacromial impingement' became both a diagnosis and an explanation for its cause, and the term is still very much alive to this day. This is despite numerous high-quality studies which have shown that this procedure, called subacromial decompression, has no better effect than exercise or sham (placebo) surgery – or indeed that the condition simply resolves itself over time – for people with subacromial-related shoulder pain. What was once one of the world's most common surgical procedures, undoubtedly helping many people, is no longer nearly as common, nor is it any longer recommended for managing shoulder pain.

WHY IS THIS STORY IMPORTANT?

If it were true that every time we lifted our arm above shoulder height, a bone spur drilled into both our bursa and rotator cuff causing shoulder pain, it would be highly unlikely that exercise would help. It would also be unlikely that symptoms would resolve on their own, and everything would point towards the need for surgical intervention to cure the condition. Such an explanatory model would therefore negatively affect our expectations towards both rehabilitation and prognosis – something we don't want. So, not only has the impingement hypothesis been thoroughly disproven as an explanation for its cause, it also puts non-surgical approaches in a very poor light.

There are several other hypotheses and theories related to subacromial shoulder pain, and what they all have in common is regarding the use, movement and loading of the arm as harmless and necessary factors for the resolution of the condition. These theories also view shoulder problems from a broader perspective, whereas 'impingement' only looks at the biomechanical causes. Today, shoulder problems are seen from a biopsychosocial perspective, where various factors from all three domains can influence pain, function and prognosis.

Although this story goes slightly beyond the purpose of this book, I believe it is important to highlight the issues related to so-called 'impingement', as it can be one of the first things that comes up when you google 'shoulder pain'.

SHOULDER PAIN

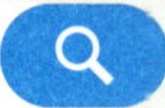

PAINFUL SHOULDERS

Painful shoulders are not, however, exclusively limited to the involvement of the rotator cuff tendons. There are several other structures in the shoulder that can contribute to the experience of shoulder pain, and currently we cannot differentiate these structures from one another in a way that allows us to definitively say, '*You have shoulder pain because of [insert structure here]*'. Therefore, rotator cuff tendinopathy falls under the umbrella term subacromial pain syndrome (SAPS), where the name suggests that all structures between the head of the humerus and the roof of the shoulder blade can be involved. This may seem confusing and frustrating, because it's natural to always want to have a definitive answer as to why we have pain in a certain area. But, on the other hand, it also gives us a great opportunity to tailor treatment. By identifying which movements and positions cause symptoms, what initially triggered the problems, and which exercises, training methods and mental strategies provide the best results for each person, most cases will resolve completely.

This section has provided an overview of shoulder injuries and problems, ranging from the specific and traumatic to the more load-related and non-specific. Different injuries and different individuals require different approaches, but what is common for all of these injuries and problems is the importance of regaining mobility, stability and strength around the shoulder. Although the shoulder may appear complex and difficult to understand, rehabilitation does not necessarily have to be difficult or complicated. However, it must be tailored to the demands that climbing as a sport places on the shoulders, while also being adapted to your characteristics as a climber.

Here are my go-to exercises for painful shoulders.

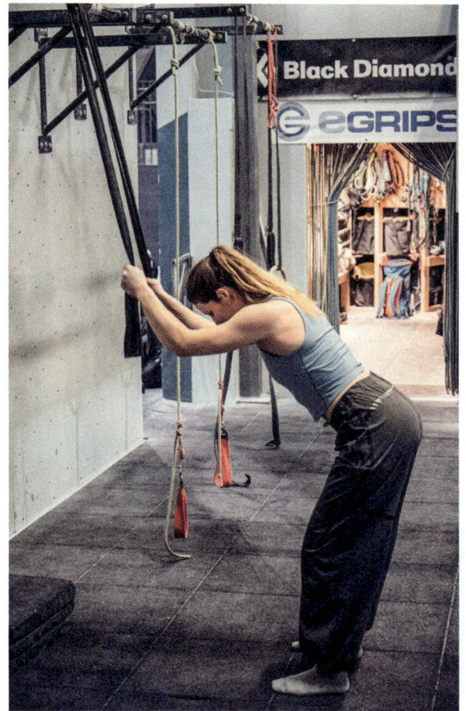

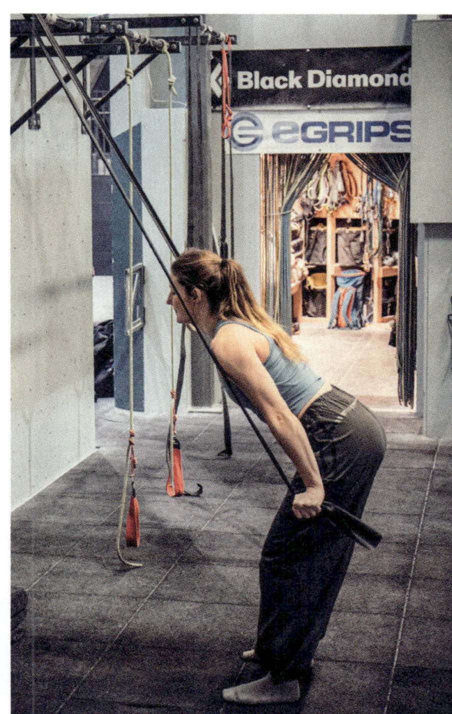

PULL-DOWNS WITH RESISTANCE BAND. This can be done as a warm-up exercise with about 20 repetitions and 2 sets, the aim of the exercise being to reduce pain when raising the arms above shoulder level.

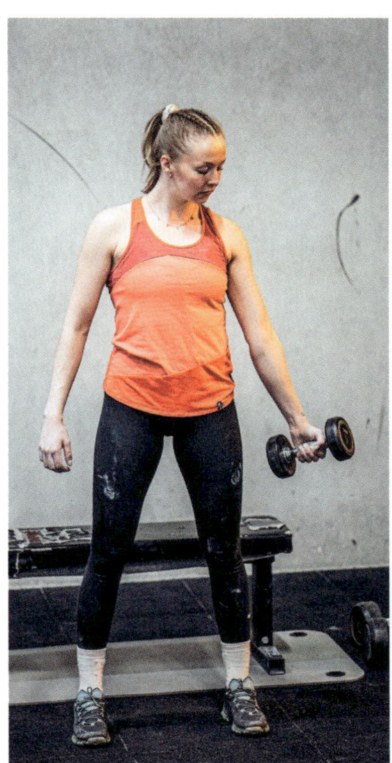

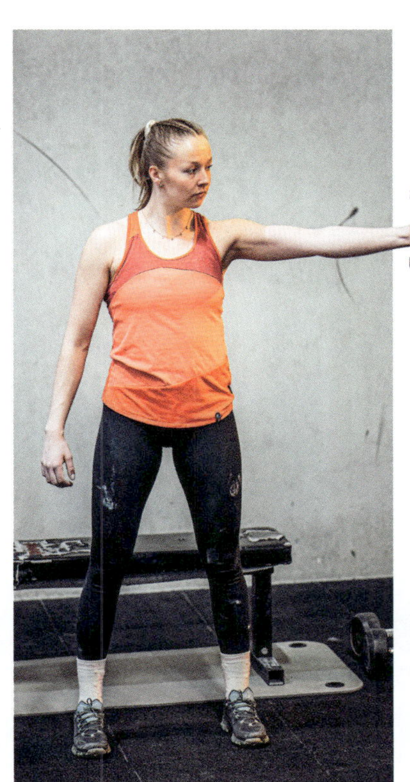

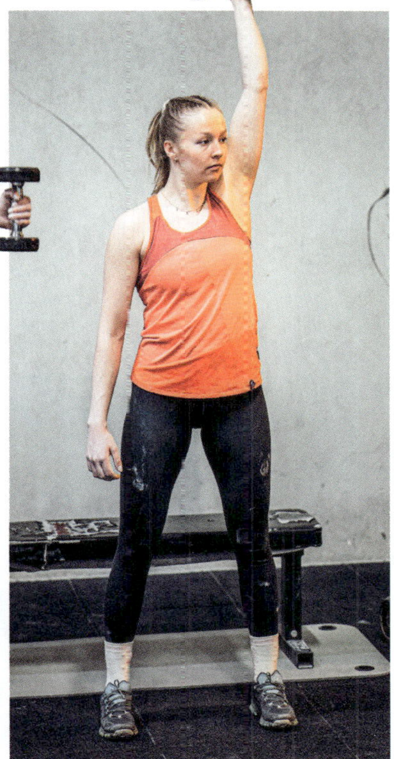

SCAPTION RAISE. Holding a dumb-bell, raise your arm out at an angle and up over your head. Do 8–10 repetitions and 2–3 sets.

EXERCISES

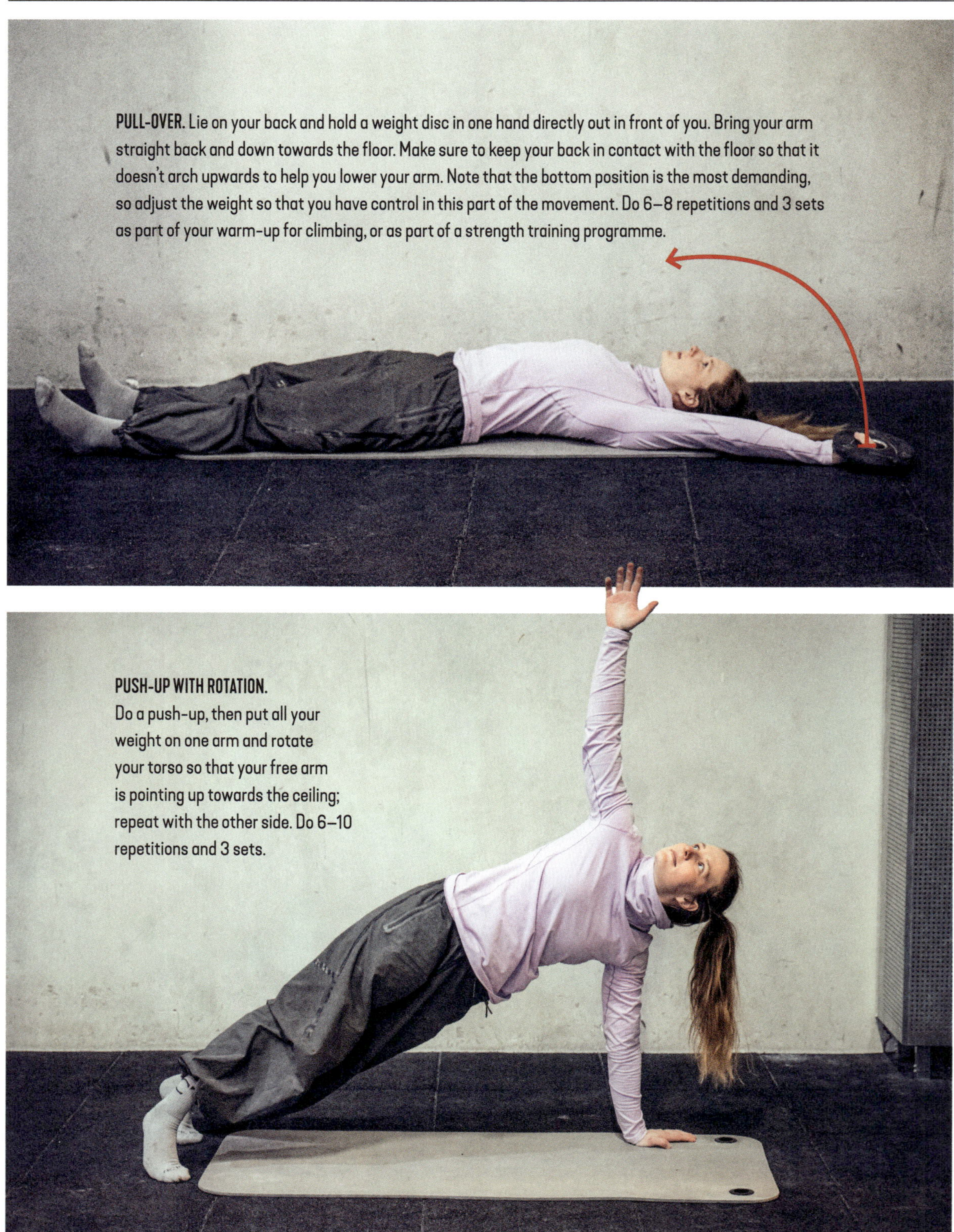

PULL-OVER. Lie on your back and hold a weight disc in one hand directly out in front of you. Bring your arm straight back and down towards the floor. Make sure to keep your back in contact with the floor so that it doesn't arch upwards to help you lower your arm. Note that the bottom position is the most demanding, so adjust the weight so that you have control in this part of the movement. Do 6–8 repetitions and 3 sets as part of your warm-up for climbing, or as part of a strength training programme.

PUSH-UP WITH ROTATION. Do a push-up, then put all your weight on one arm and rotate your torso so that your free arm is pointing up towards the ceiling; repeat with the other side. Do 6–10 repetitions and 3 sets.

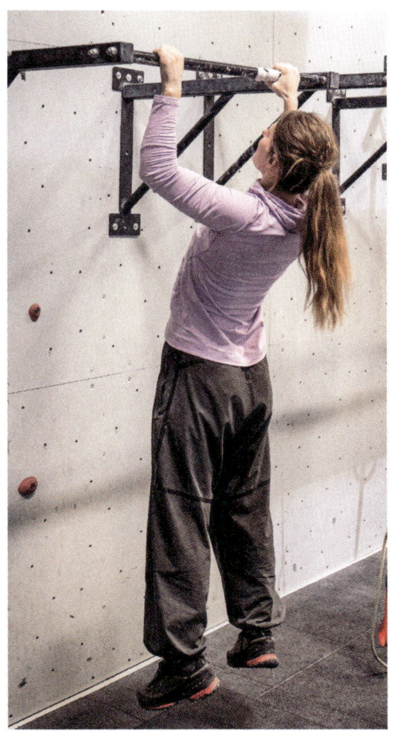

MID-RANGE PULL-UP. It's usually the bottom position, and in some cases the top position, that is troublesome. So, the solution for training strength can be to train in the so-called 'mid-range', i.e. avoiding the outer positions, but training heavily in the part of the movement path that is symptom-free.

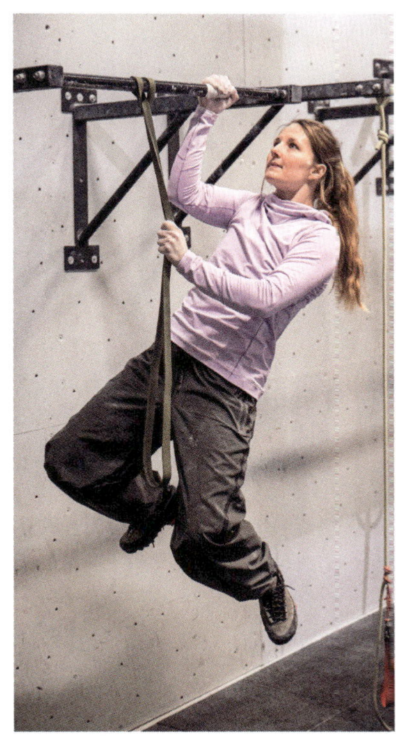

ASSISTED ONE-ARM LOCK-OFF. Do 2 hangs of 10 seconds at both 90 degrees and 135 degrees of elbow flexion.

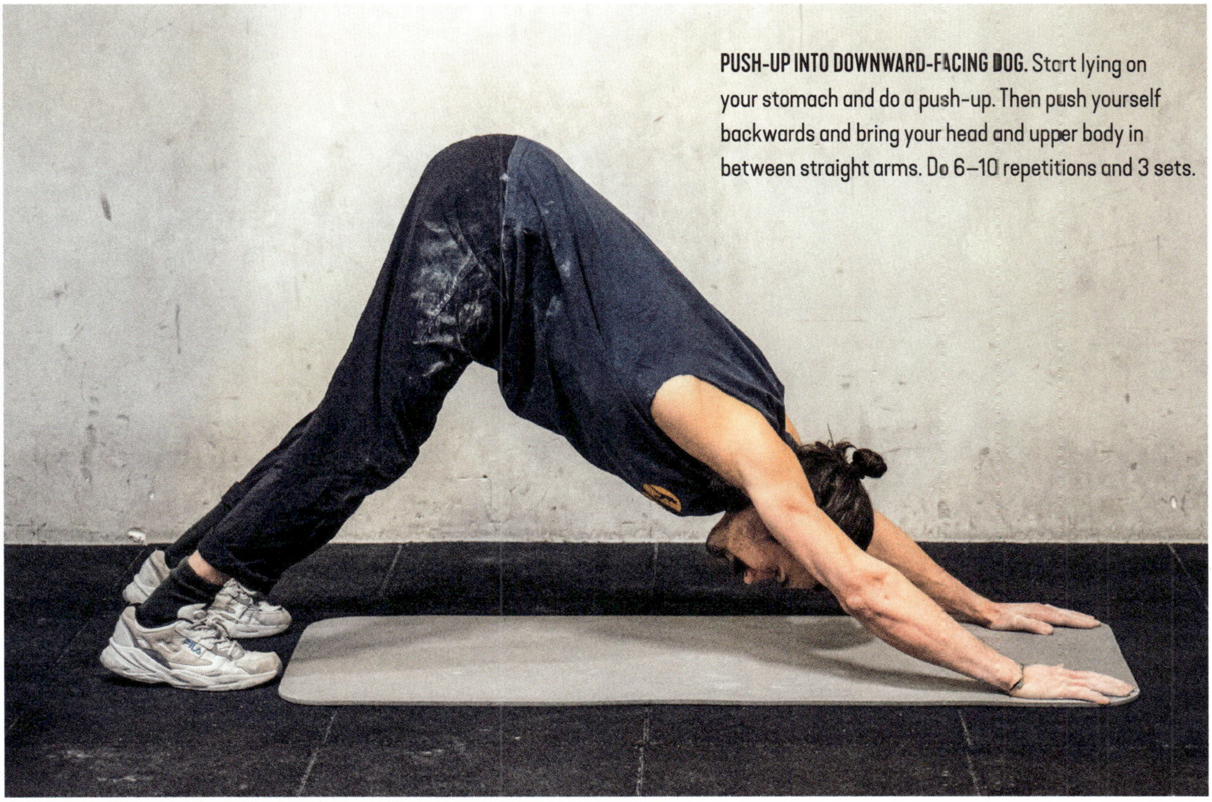

PUSH-UP INTO DOWNWARD-FACING DOG. Start lying on your stomach and do a push-up. Then push yourself backwards and bring your head and upper body in between straight arms. Do 6–10 repetitions and 3 sets.

KNEES AND THIGHS

MENISCI, COLLATERAL LIGAMENTS AND CRUCIATE LIGAMENTS

Climbing knee injuries that are not caused by falls are on the rise, and certain climbing positions and movements stand out as triggers: high steps/rockovers, drop knees and heel hooks. What these positions have in common is a bend in the knee with the shin rotated outwards. And the more bending and rotation, the more stress that is placed on the stabilising structures of the knee joint: menisci, collateral ligaments and cruciate ligaments. We usually use these climbing positions and movements when handholds, body positions and moves require us to take the strain off the fingers and relieve the upper body as much as possible. For example, we perform a rockover when the handholds are poor or far apart, moving our centre of gravity to maintain balance or move towards the next grip. The knee is then maximally bent with an externally rotated leg, while we try to straighten the leg to reach for the next hold. A similar knee position can be seen during a drop-knee manoeuvre. Both positions exert immense pressure on the menisci and the medial collateral ligament. A heel hook can be performed at various knee angles, but they typically involve an externally rotated shin with a strong pull from the hamstring muscles to flex the knee. This places a high load on the knee joint overall, but it particularly stresses the menisci and the lateral collateral ligament.

Acute knee injuries usually result in pain and swelling, which limits mobility and function. It's important to clinically examine the knee to assess whether imaging is needed. While ultrasound can detect fluid in the joint and injuries to the collateral ligaments, MRI is necessary for evaluating whether any meniscal or cruciate ligament injuries should be treated surgically. In cases where there is pronounced swelling or locking of the knee joint – i.e. an inability to move it – one should seek medical attention promptly and undergo evaluation for possible surgical treatment.

Can non-fall-related knee injuries be prevented? Well, we can at least reduce the risk by being aware of the positions that push the knee joint to its limits and making a cost-benefit assessment. Some routes and boulders have moves where we simply cannot avoid a high rockover, a deep drop knee, or an awkward heel hook or heel-toe cam. In such cases, we must consider whether we're willing to take the risk. Perhaps we are willing to risk it on a project, but not during our training sessions. This approach will drastically reduce the number of times the knee is in a vulnerable position, which also reduces the risk of injury. However, we also lose the opportunity to train these positions, which is important for both mastering them technically and being better prepared for encountering them on future projects.

Therefore, my suggestion is to practise rockovers, drop knees and heel hooks as part of your technical training – either in separate sessions or as part of your warm-up exercises. This way, you can use better handholds and footholds to control the load on your knee joint and gradually make it more resilient to higher loads in vulnerable positions.

EXERCISES

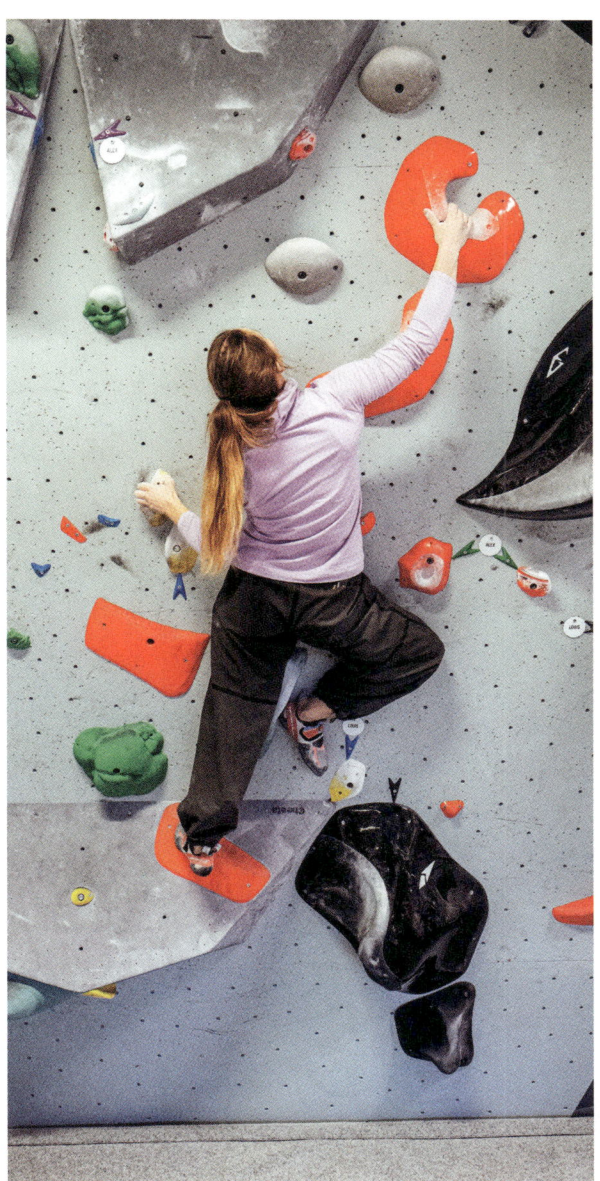

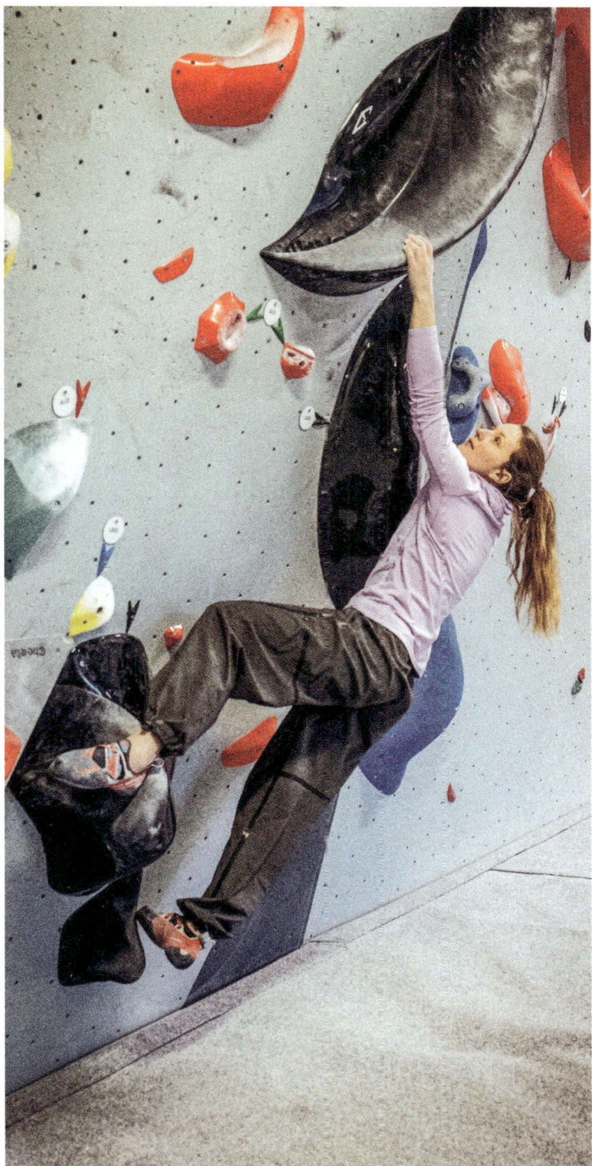

Heel hooks at different knee angles and with varying degrees of leg rotation.

EXERCISES

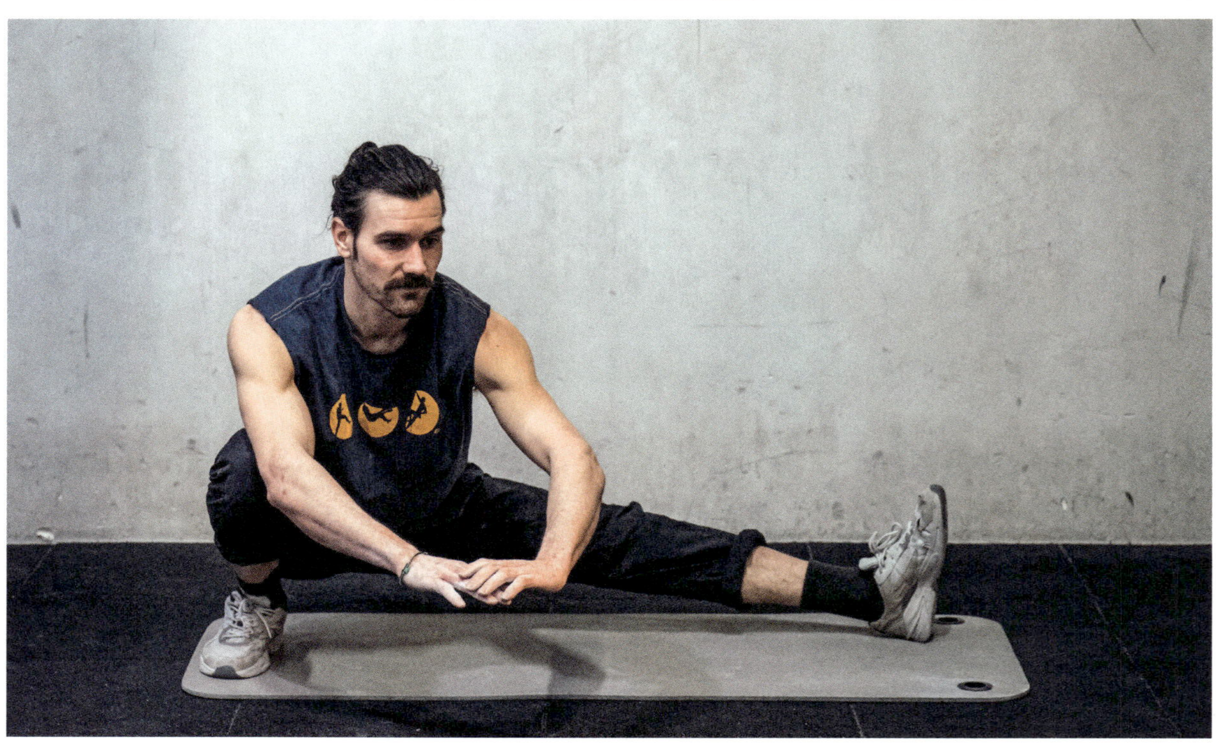

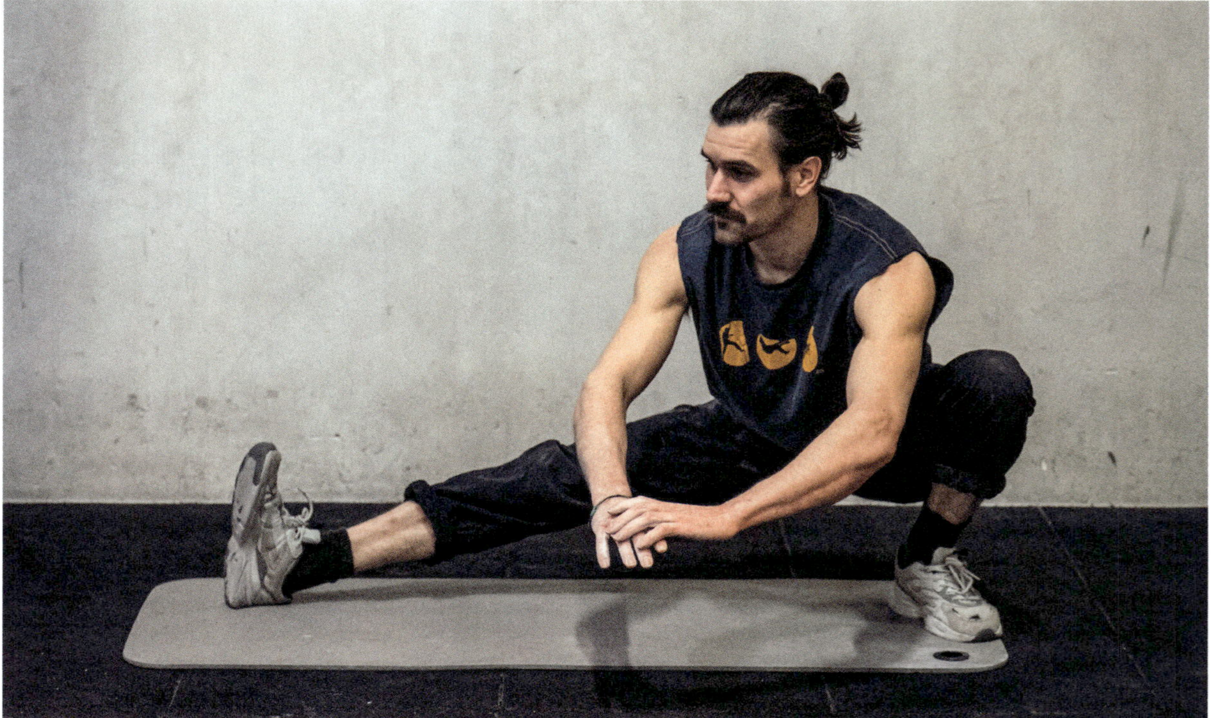

COSSACK SQUAT. Start standing with legs apart. Sit down over one foot while keeping the other leg straight. Stand up and repeat on the opposite side. Perform 8–10 repetitions and 2 sets.

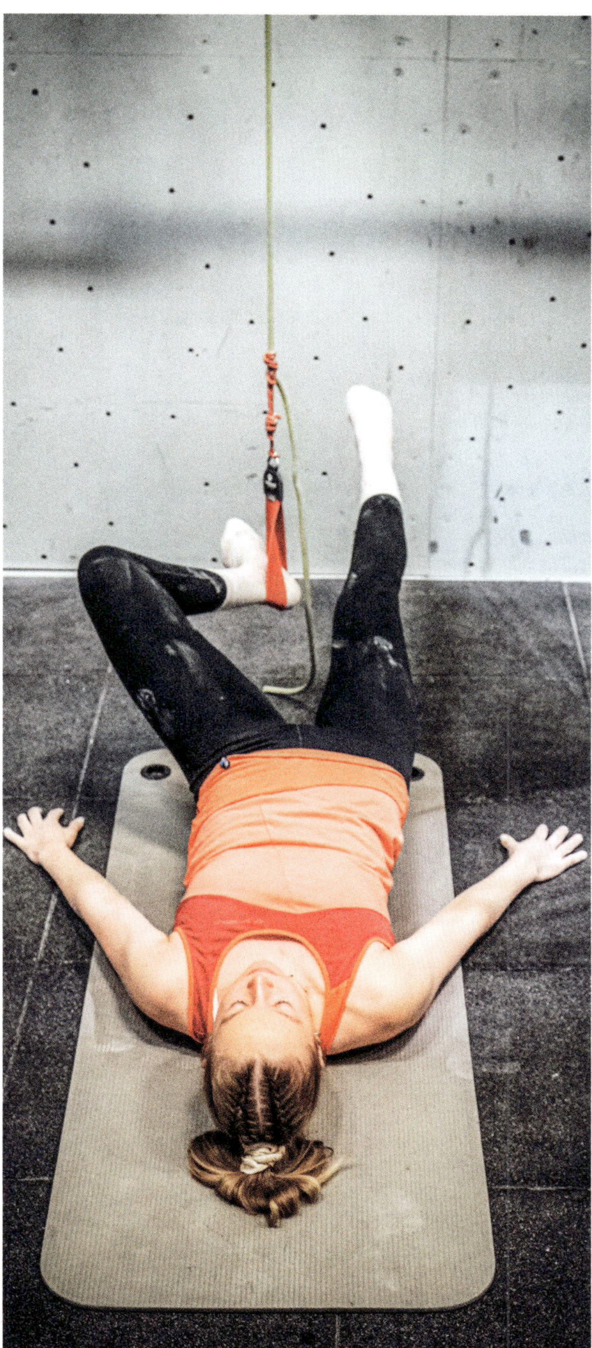

BRIDGE AND PULL IN. By placing the heel in a sling and rotating the leg outwards, you can lift your body off the ground and simulate the load in a heel hook. Press the outside of your heel into the sling, lift your body and pull your leg towards you so that your knee is at a 90-degree angle. Perform 6 repetitions and 2 sets.

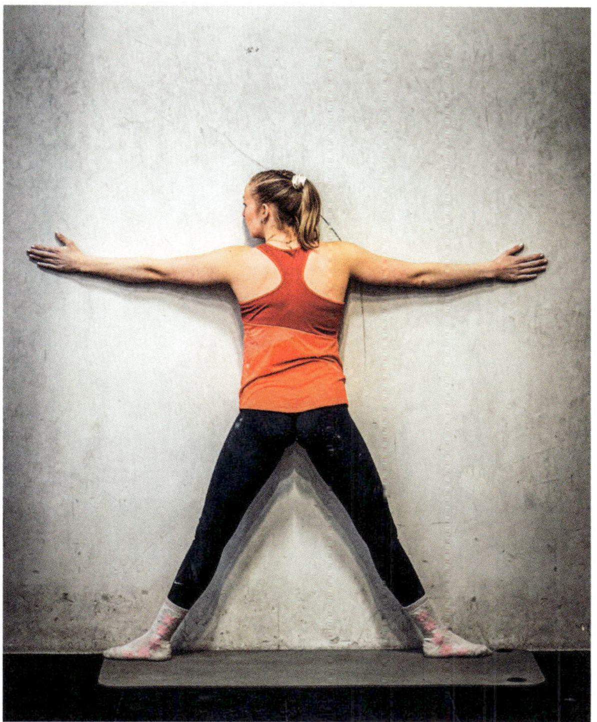

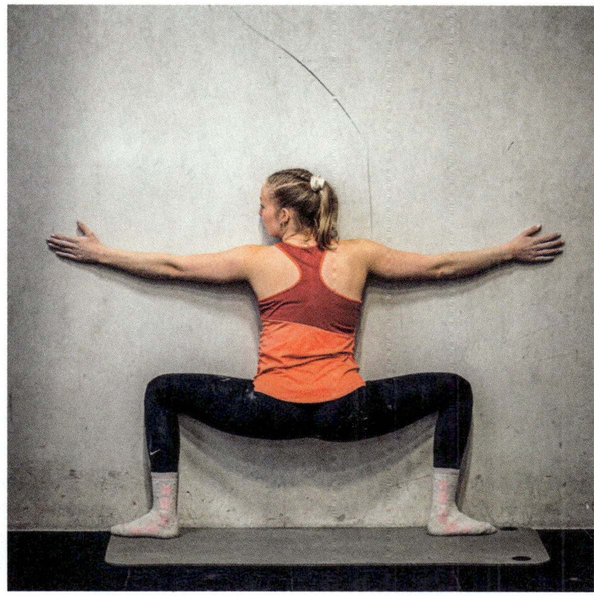

WALL SQUAT. This is an exercise to simulate high foot movements and rockovers, where you need to rotate your hips and calves and push yourself up from a deep position. Start standing and slowly lower yourself as far down as you can while maintaining contact between the wall and your knees and upper body. Perform 8–10 repetitions and 2 sets.

HAMSTRING INJURIES

'I went for a heel hook and felt a jerk in the back of my thigh, almost up to my butt. Now it hurts when I walk and straighten my knee. I haven't even dared to think about heel hooks and climbing.'

The hamstring is a group of three muscles at the back of the thigh. They extend at the hip joint, flex at the knee joint and rotate the shin bone inwards or outwards in relation to the thigh bone, and are susceptible to strains in the whole muscle-tendon-bone unit during heel hooks and the splits.

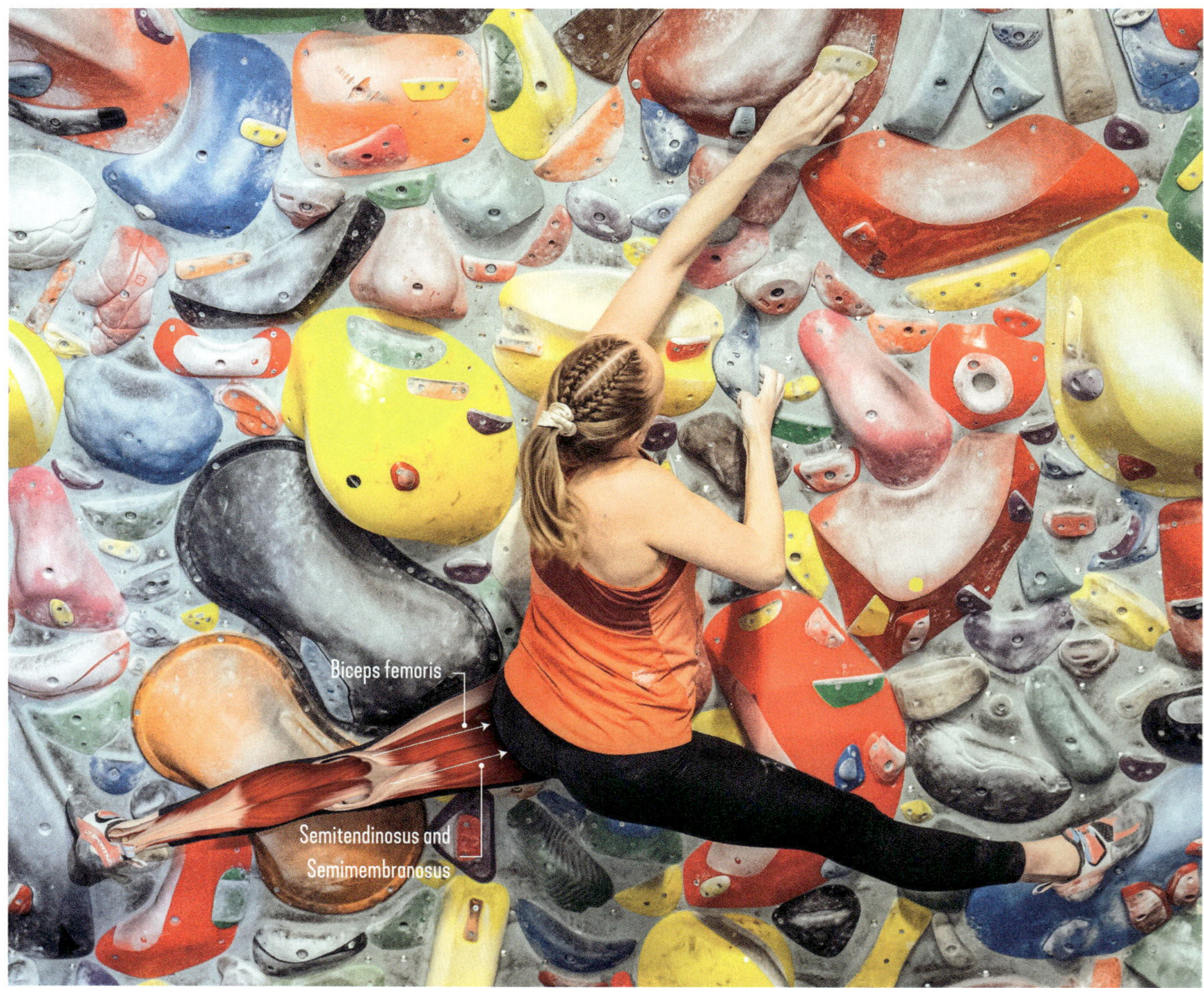

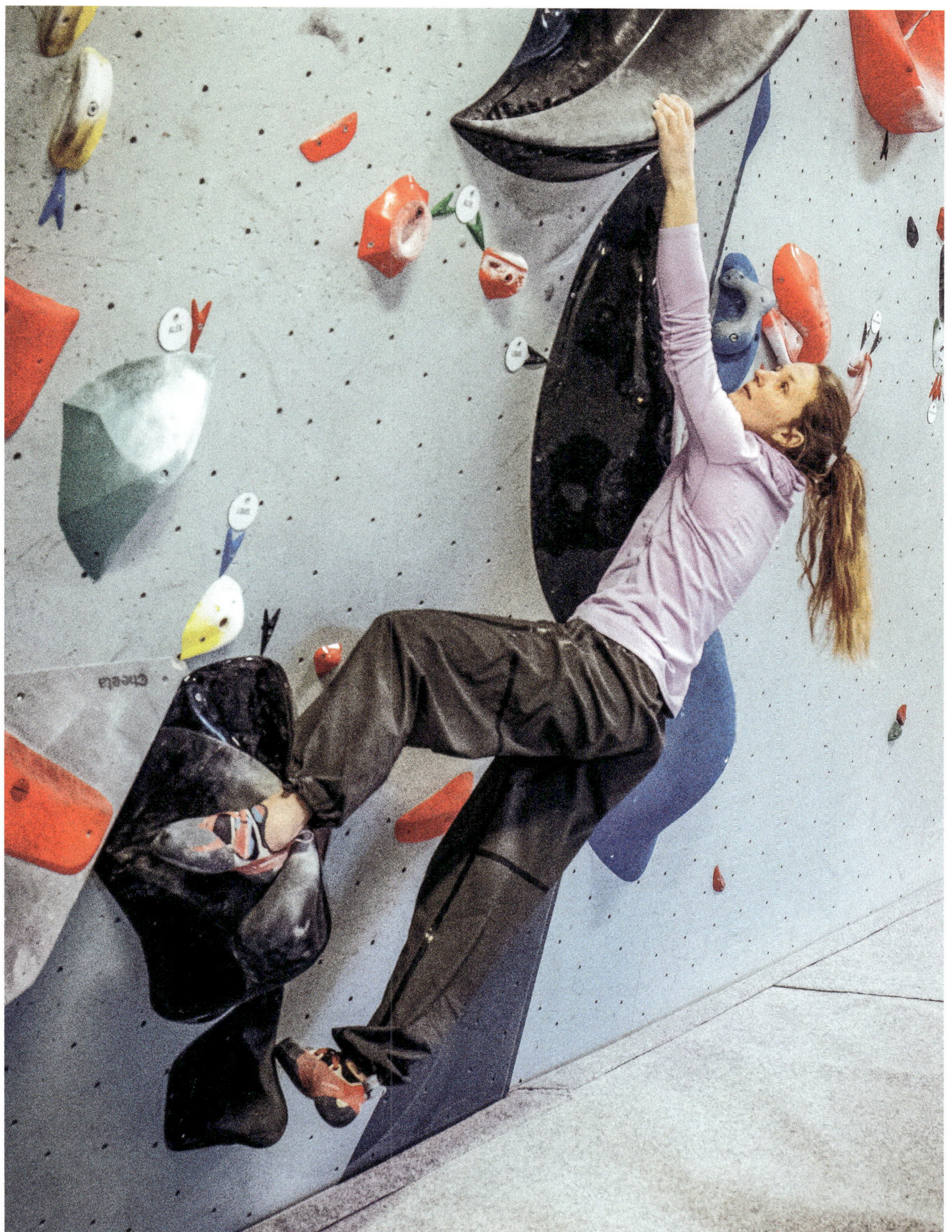

By pressing the heel against the foothold, the leg muscles contract to either hold the body in one position or pull it towards the next handhold.

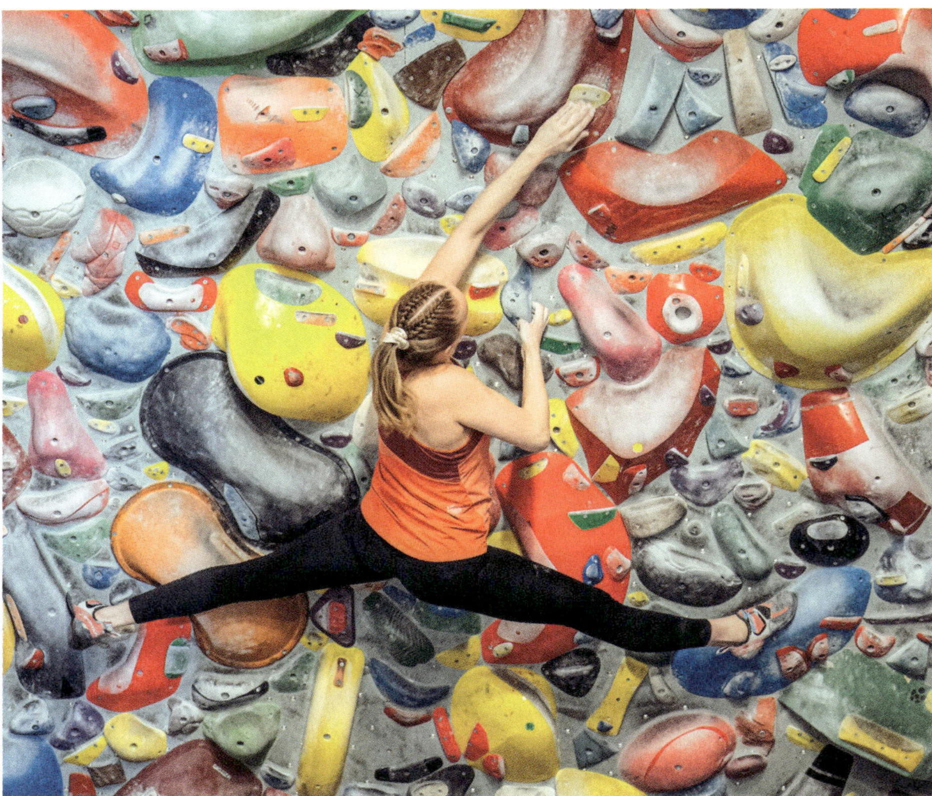

In a split, the hamstrings must contract to maintain the extended position.

Hamstring injuries are classified based on their location: either at the knee or at the hip. Injuries in the knee region are generally located to the back and outer side of the knee, where the tendons from the biceps femoris muscle attach to the fibula. Injuries in the hip region are mostly located close the sitting bone, where the majority of the hamstring muscles attach to the pelvis.

While the mechanisms for these two types of injuries have been well documented in running-based sports, they have been explored far less in climbing. We assume that hip-related injuries occur during close-in heel hooks, which involve a high degree of hip flexion. More open hip positions – when the hip isn't bent as much while pulling on a heel and we simultaneously rotate the shin bone outwards for maximum pressure on our heel – predispose us more towards knee-related injuries. These are acute injuries and many climbers will experience a tearing or popping at the back of their thigh.

Strains involving both muscles and tendons should be examined thoroughly to assess the degree and extent of the injury (see table on page 71 regarding the grading of injuries). In most cases, the approach to treatment will involve a temporary cessation of hamstring-related movements and a gradual rehabilitation, but with more extensive tendon tears, or a tearing of the tendon attachment itself, surgery may be necessary. Therefore, it is my recommendation that all acute hamstring injuries should be examined by a healthcare professional so that a course of action can be determined as quickly as possible.

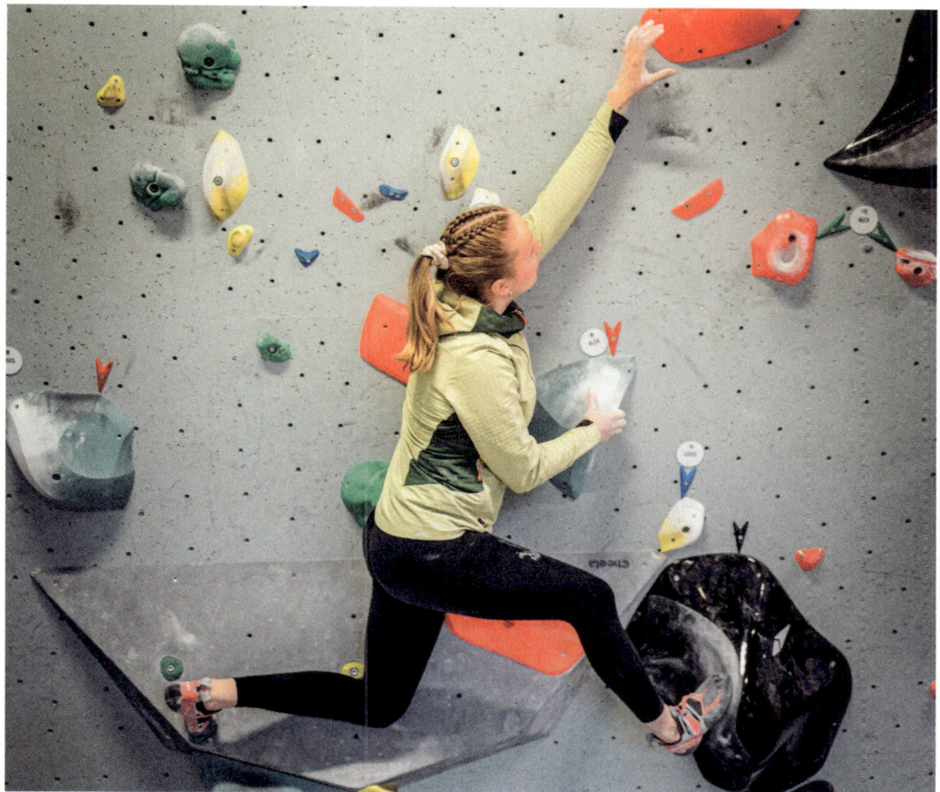

In a drop-knee, the hamstring muscles work to help maintain contact with the footholds and to keep the hips close to the wall.

Uzo Ehiogu and colleagues published an article in 2020 which advocated for an alternative management approach for hamstring injuries in climbers compared with hamstring injuries in runners and sprinters. They argued that while running-related sports aim to strengthen the hamstrings through extension – eccentric training – the biomechanics of climbing are the opposite. We must instead strengthen our hamstrings isometrically and concentrically to meet the demands posed by heel hooking. This does not exclude eccentric training of the hamstrings, but emphasises that we must train in a climbing-specific manner.

A rehabilitation plan for hamstring injuries goes through various phases with different goals, representing the different requirements for both the muscle-tendon unit and the entire kinetic chain. In our case as climbers, this involves training the hamstrings in various ways from the time of injury until full recovery, as well as building capacity in the fingers, arms, upper body and core. This latter capacity is often underemphasised, but it's obvious that stronger fingers, arms, upper body and core can give us the ability to relieve the stress on our hamstrings during demanding heel hook positions. The rehabilitation process should therefore focus on becoming a stronger and better climber from a holistic perspective, rather than just training the hamstring muscles in isolation.

MOBILITY EXERCISES

The first stage of rehabilitation after a strain injury is aimed at stretching the muscles.

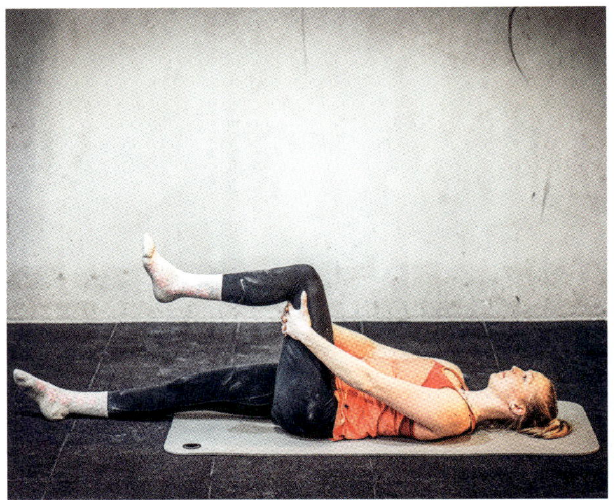

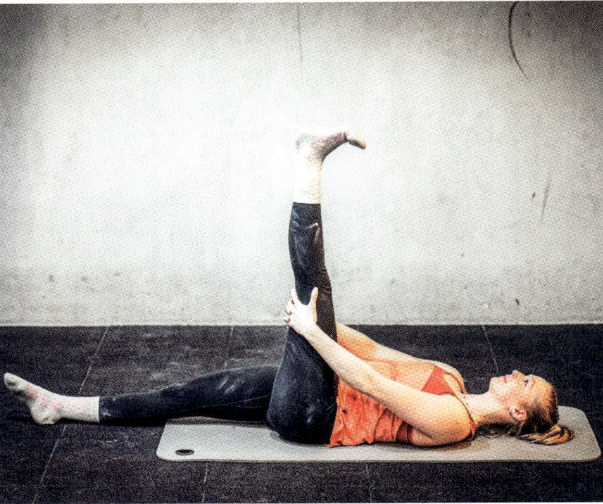

EXERCISE 1: EXTENDER. Hold your leg behind your knee and straighten your leg as far as you can. Do 12–15 repetitions and 2 sets, daily.

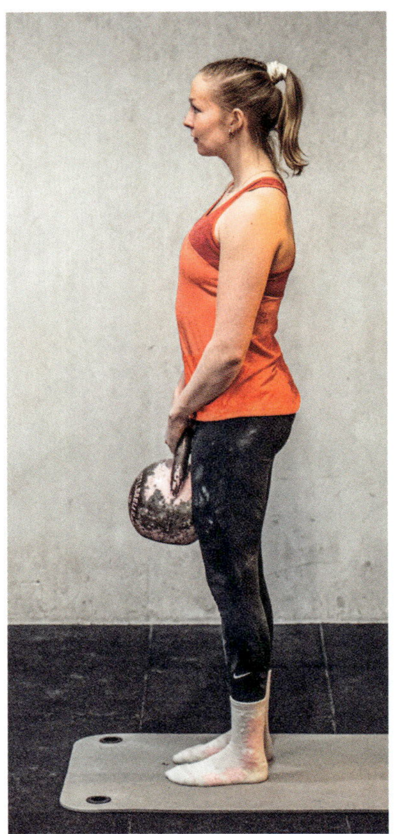

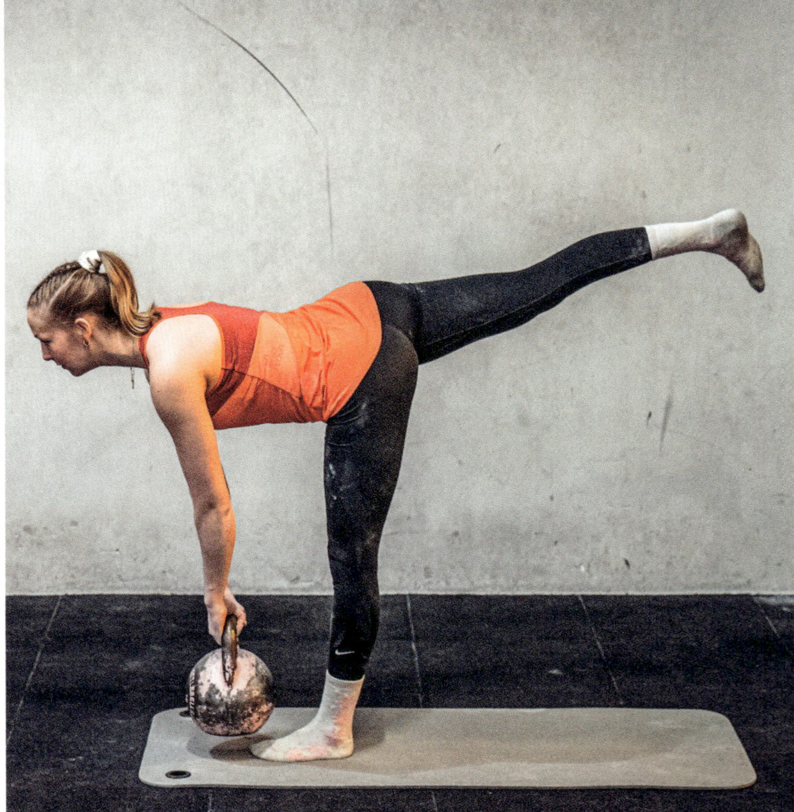

EXERCISE 2: DIVER. Stand on one leg and bring your upper body straight forwards while straightening your back leg. Start with no weight to begin with and then add weight gradually as you can go deeper into the position. Do 6 repetitions and 3 sets every other day.

The next stage of rehab aims to load the muscles in different ways.

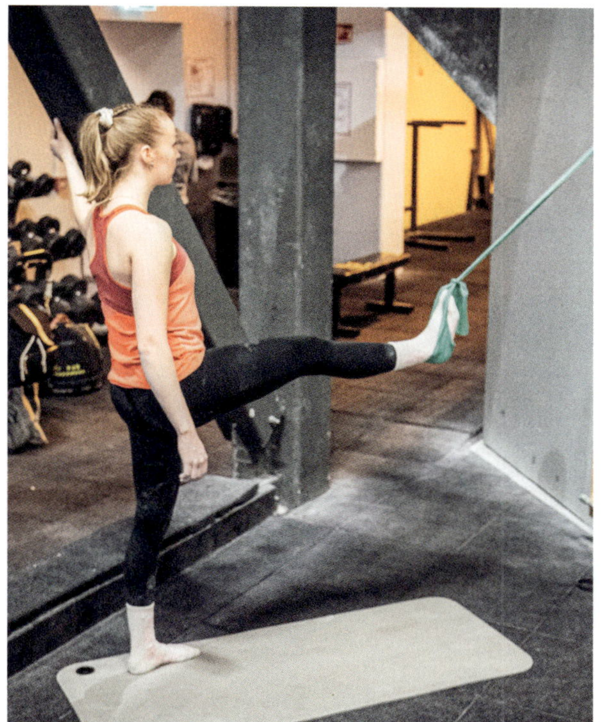

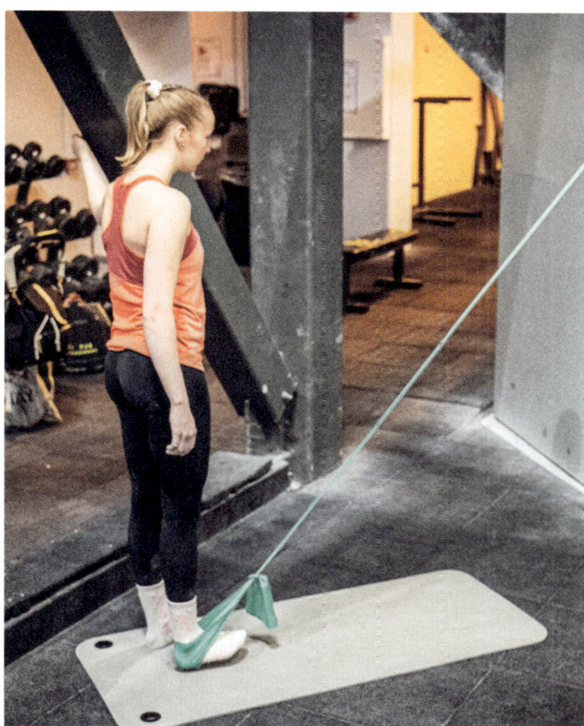

STRAIGHT HIP EXTENSION. With your leg held out in front of you and with a resistance band around your ankle, move your leg down and back until it is parallel with your standing leg. Do 12 repetitions and 3 sets, twice a week.

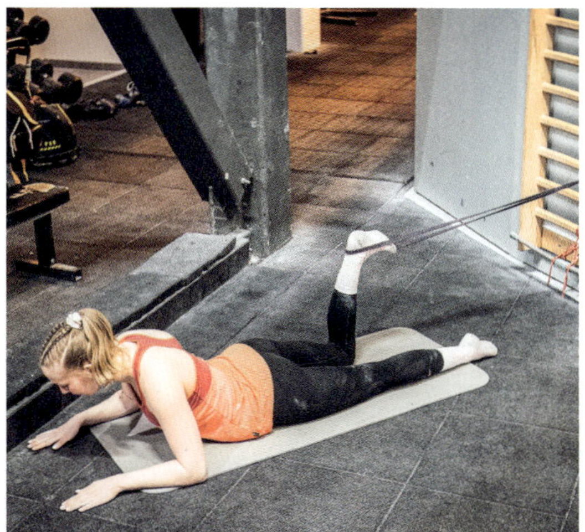

LEG CURLS. Lie on your stomach with the resistance band around your ankle, and bend your knee so that your heel moves back towards your body. Do 12 repetitions and 3 sets, twice a week.

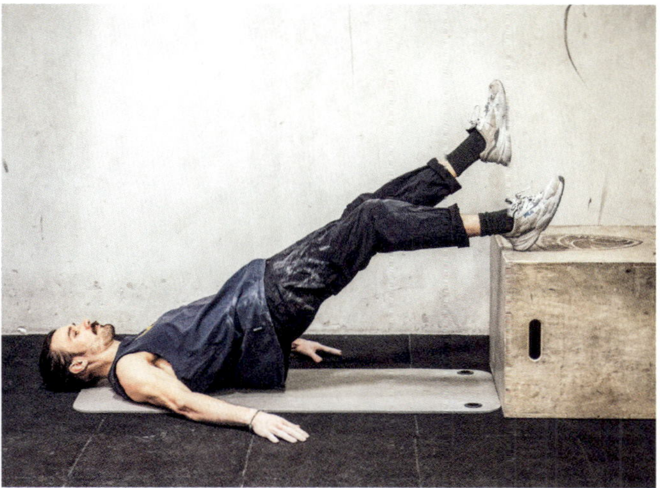

SINGLE-LEG BRIDGE. Start lying on your back with one leg on a box, crash pad or similar. Press your heel against the surface and lift your body off the floor. Vary the angle of your knee and how far you turn your leg out to the side. Do 12 repetitions and 3 sets, twice a week.

EXERCISES

HEAVY, SLOW STRENGTH TRAINING

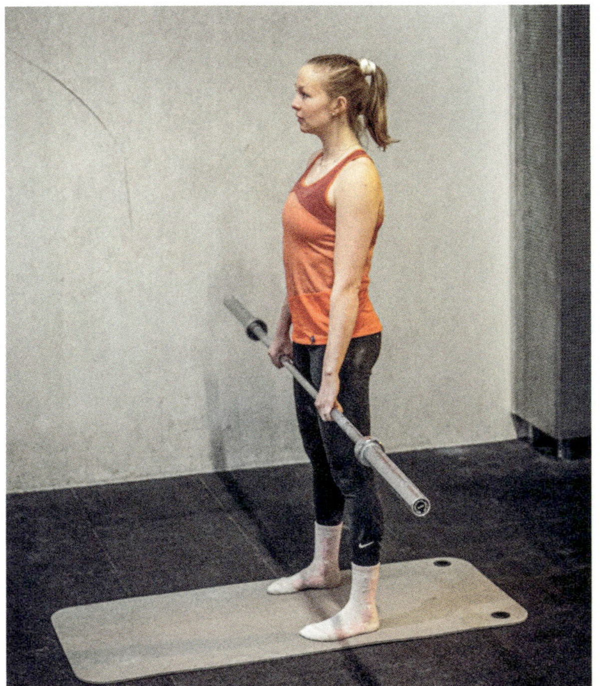

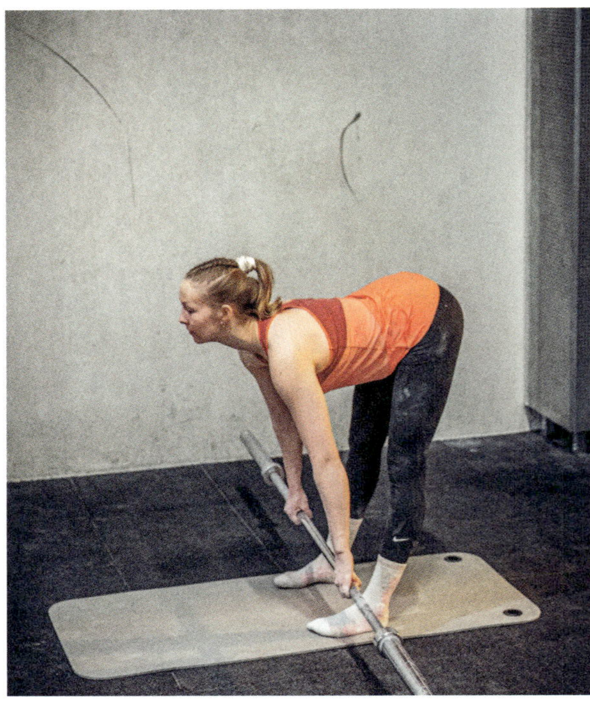

STRAIGHT DEADLIFT. Holding a barbell, drop your upper body forwards while keeping your legs straight. Tighten the backs of your thighs and lift your upper body back to the starting position. Perform for 6 repetitions and 3 sets, twice a week.

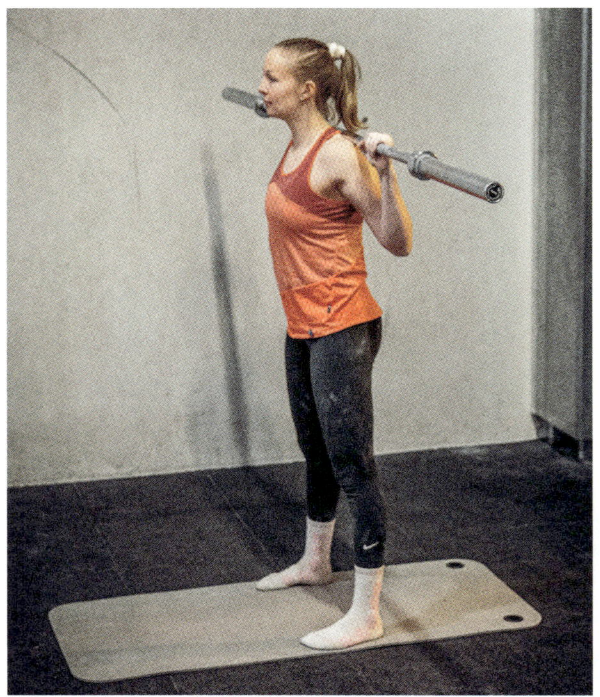

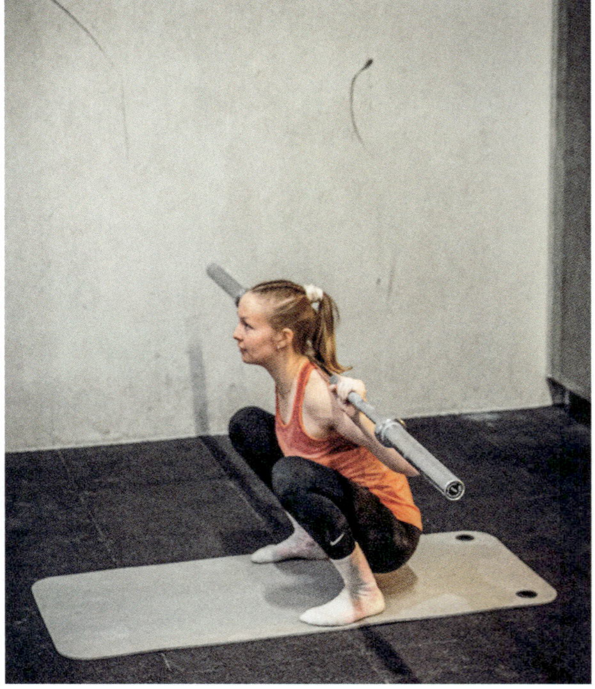

DEEP SQUAT. With a barbell on your back, squat down and stand up again. Note that this is a demanding position for the knee joints, so take this into account when determining the weight you use for the exercise. Perform 6 repetitions and 3 sets, twice a week.

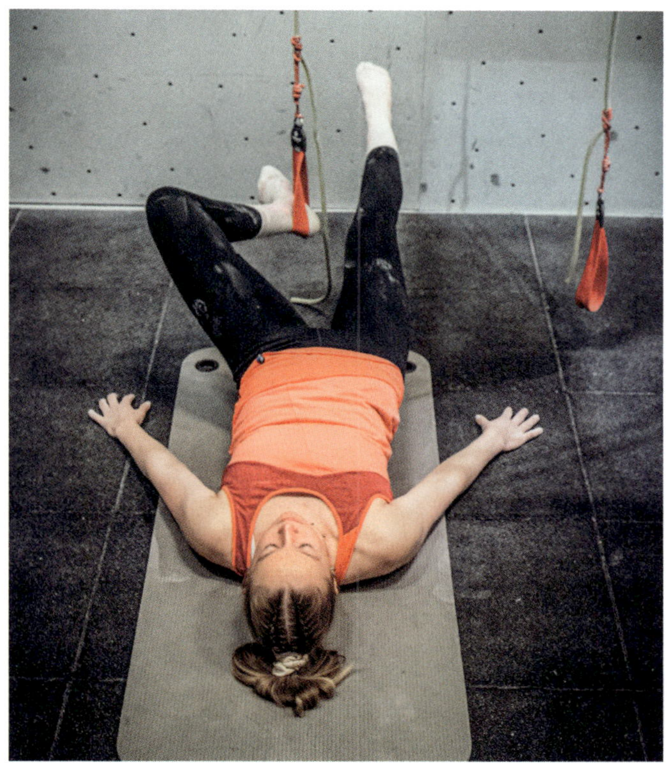

BRIDGE AND PULL IN. Press the outside of your heel into the sling, lift your body and pull your leg towards you so that your knee is at a 90-degree angle. Perform 6 repetitions and 3 sets, twice a week.

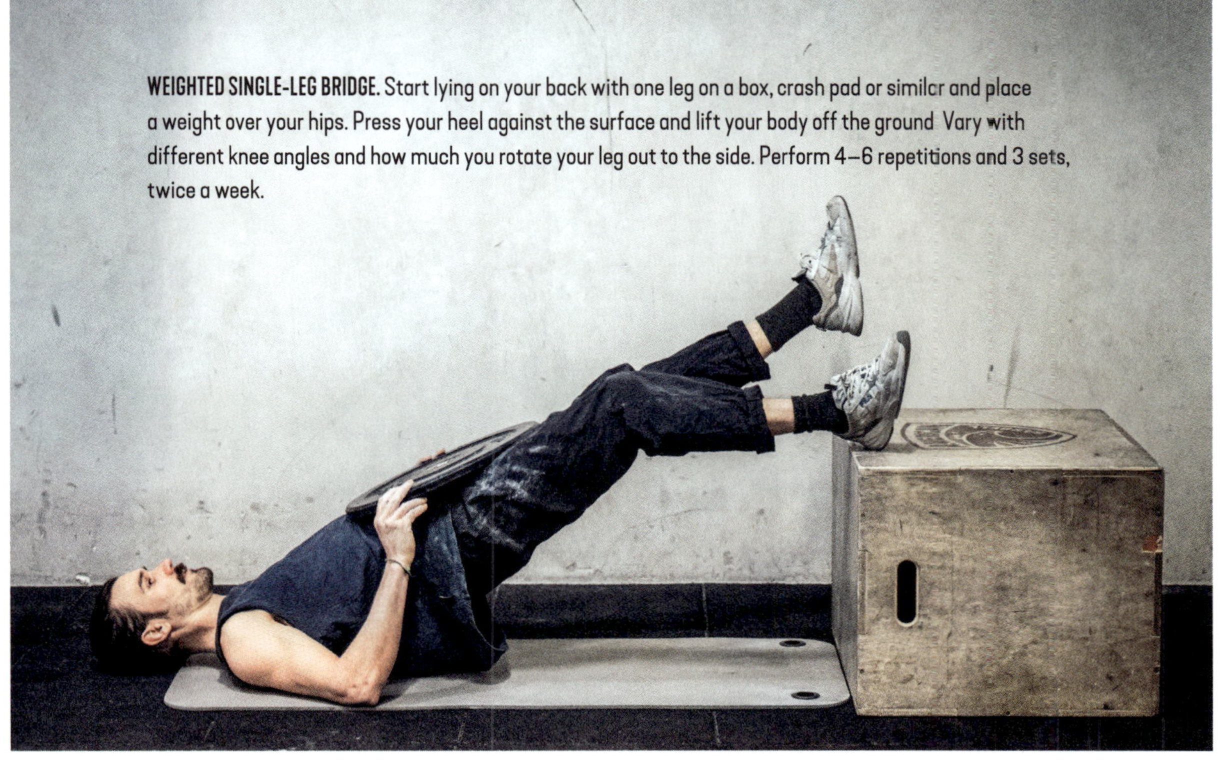

WEIGHTED SINGLE-LEG BRIDGE. Start lying on your back with one leg on a box, crash pad or similar and place a weight over your hips. Press your heel against the surface and lift your body off the ground. Vary with different knee angles and how much you rotate your leg out to the side. Perform 4–6 repetitions and 3 sets, twice a week.

ANKLE SPRAINS

'I missed the pad a bit and landed wrong. My ankle swelled up almost immediately, and I had to be helped out of the forest and back to the car. It hurts to put weight on my foot, and the ankle feels stiff. What do I do now?'

I've had this phone call quite a few times. I've also been on the other end of the line, having landed all wrong and sprained my own ankle, so knowing how to handle an ankle sprain is good knowledge to have. As with all acute injuries, you should follow PEACE & LOVE (see pages 18–19), where Protection, Elevation and Compression are most important in the initial phase when you get off the pad and into your car to go home. This means: stop climbing, wrap a compression bandage around your ankle and try to keep your leg elevated above heart level. This lowers the risk of worsening the injury and reduces the swelling around the ankle.

The next step is to rule out a fracture. Sometimes, it's (unfortunately) easy to detect a fracture, but smaller fractures may not be visible to the naked eye. In such cases, you can use the Ottawa ankle rules (opposite), combined with an assessment of whether or not you can bear full body weight on the injured ankle. If there's any suspicion of a possible fracture, it's advisable to visit a hospital for an X-ray so that you're not walking around on a fracture that needs offloading and proper rest for optimal healing.

If it's not a fracture, though, the recommendation is to resume weight bearing within the first 48 hours. This doesn't mean limping around; crutches can be used if needed while moving from point A to point B, but do practise putting some weight on your leg without limping when taking single steps. Since swelling and pain limit mobility in the ankle joint, active exercises should be initiated early in order to increase the range of motion and stimulate muscles. Even if there's some pain during the exercises, it's important to pay greater attention to the swelling afterwards: gravity alone will cause the ankle to swell up after you've been walking around compared to when it has been elevated above heart level, but the training itself should not lead to an increase in swelling.

A swollen ankle has poorer joint proprioception and thus poorer stability, increasing the risk of re-injury from a premature return to activities that demand high ankle function. Therefore, you should progress slowly from weight-bearing and simple exercises, towards being able to jump and land on the foot and making quick changes in direction before you return to full sporting activity. It's easy to think that the ankle isn't so important for us climbers, but anyone who's sprained their ankle knows how inhibiting it is to climb with a stiff and painful ankle. So, even though it's quickly possible to start top-roping again, I recommend specifically training an ankle for five minutes a day, five days a week for five weeks after a sprain. This way you'll regain strength, mobility and stability, and you'll be able to take falls both on lead and while bouldering, while also regaining confidence in your ankle in all of the movements and positions it is exposed to on the wall.

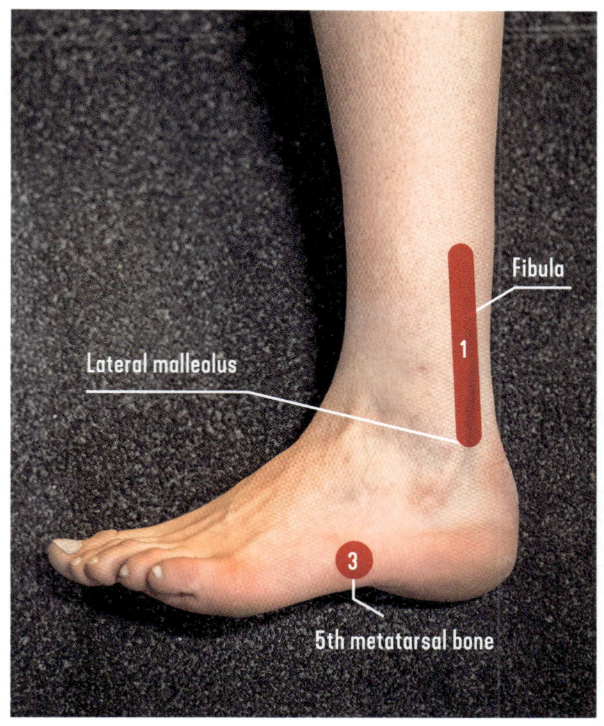

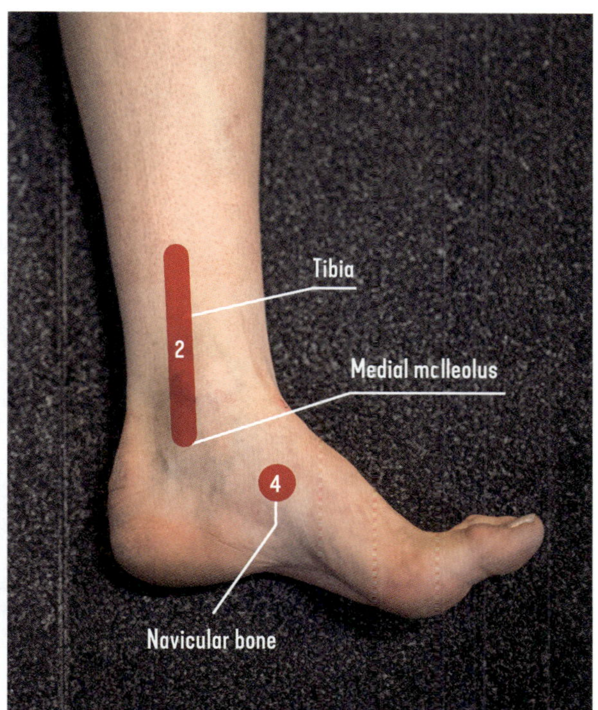

OTTAWA ANKLE RULES:

1. Bony tenderness along distal 6cm of the posterior edge of fibula or tip of lateral malleolus.
2. Bony tenderness along distal 6cm of the posterior edge of tibia or tip of medial malleolus.
3. Bony tenderness at the base of the 5th metatarsal bone.
4. Bony tenderness at the navicular bone.
5. Inability to bear weight both immediately after injury and for 4 steps during initial examination.

If pain over the ankle bones plus 1, 2 or 5, X-ray of the ankle is recommended.
If pain over the midfoot plus 3, 4 or 5, X-ray of the foot is recommended.
A score of 0 out of 5 indicates less than a 1 per cent probability of fracture.

EXERCISES

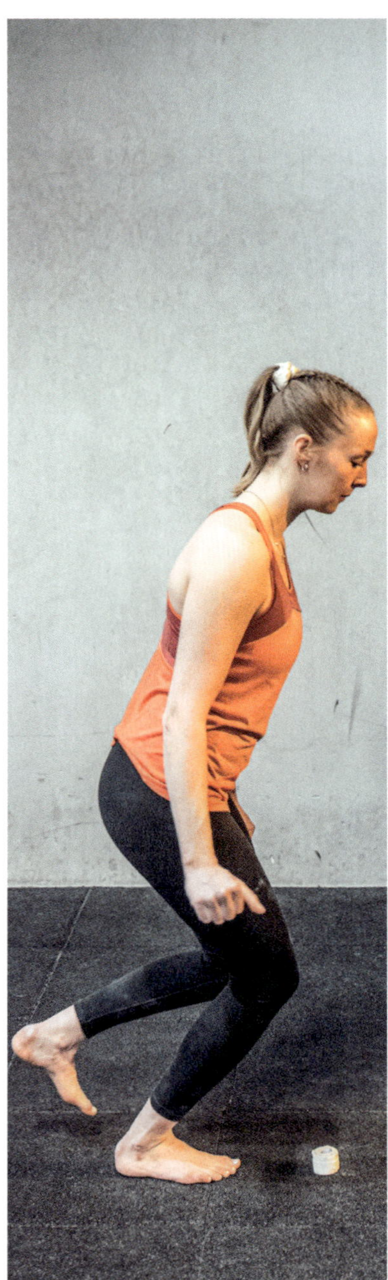

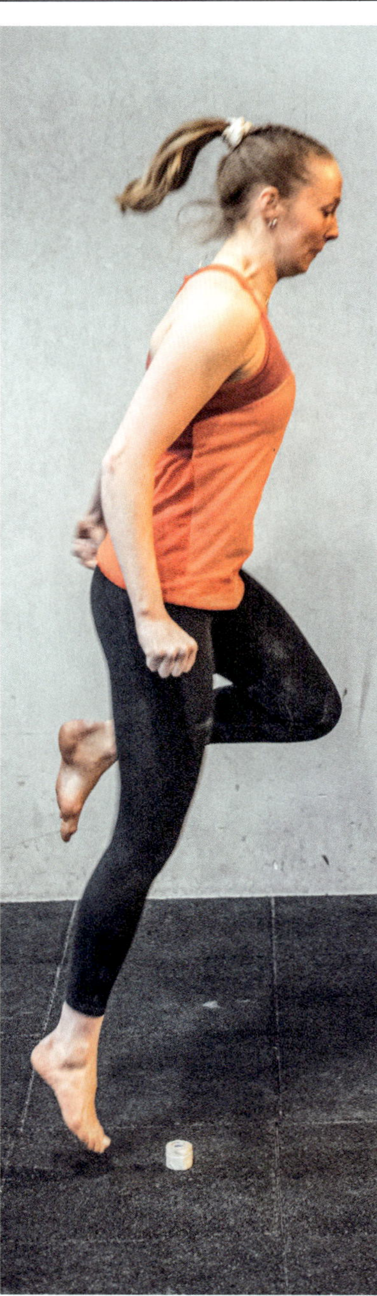

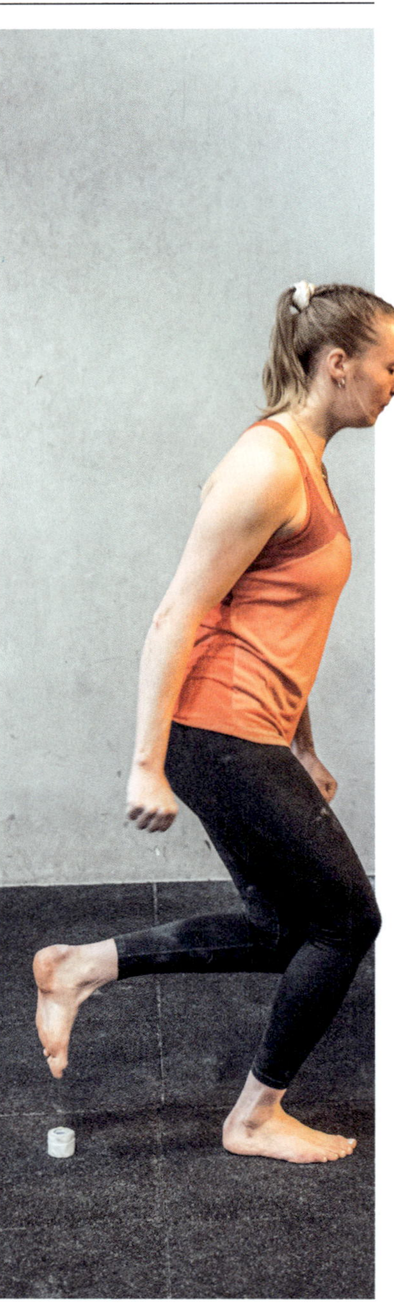

HOPPING EXERCISES. Your imagination is the only limit to what you can eventually do! Practising take-offs and landings will help you react faster and stabilise your ankle better in the event of a fall, and it's easy to include such exercises as part of your warm-up for a climbing session. Then you can hop forwards, backwards, sideways, in star formation, and up and down from boxes. Do 6–12 hops per set, and do 3 sets per session.

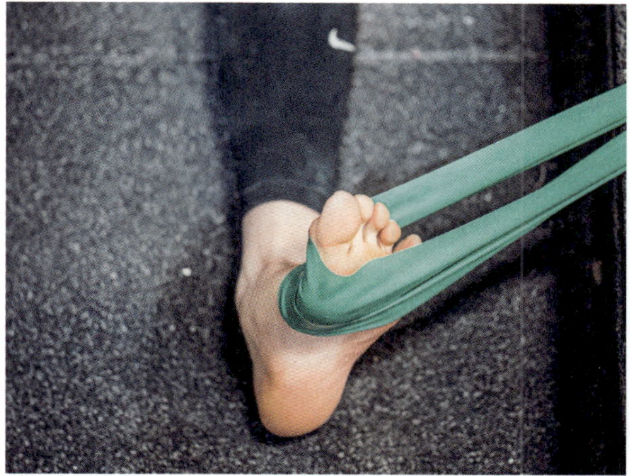

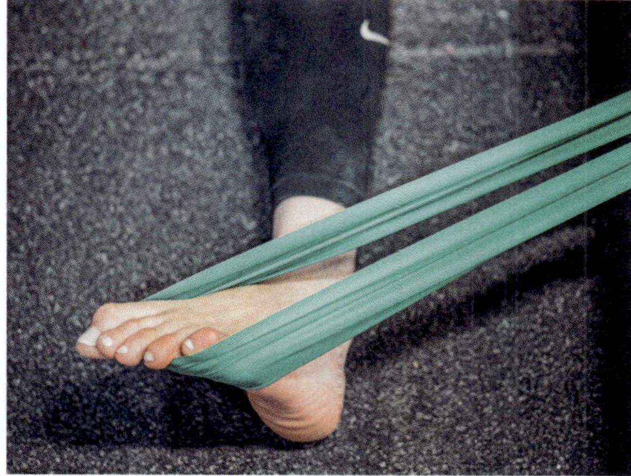

Wrap a wide resistance band around the inside of your foot and rotate your foot inwards. Do 12–15 repetitions, twice a day.

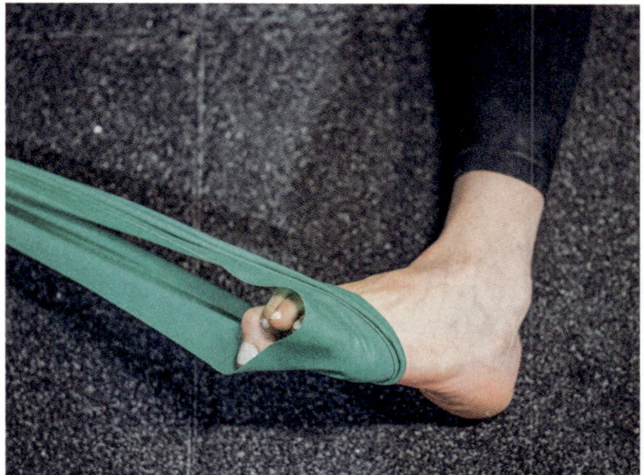

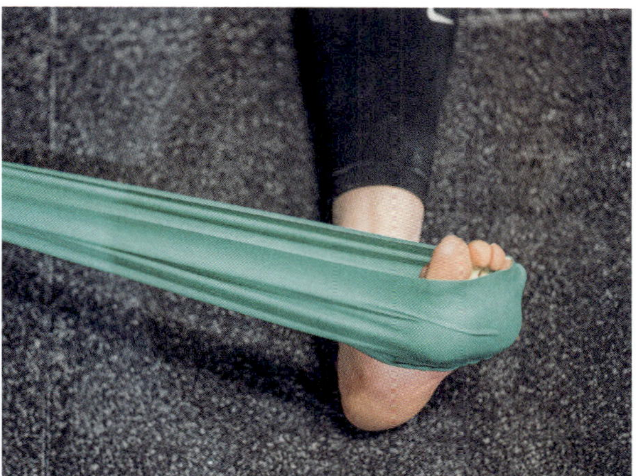

Wrap a wide resistance band around the outside of your foot and rotate your foot outwards. Do 12–15 repetitions, twice a day.

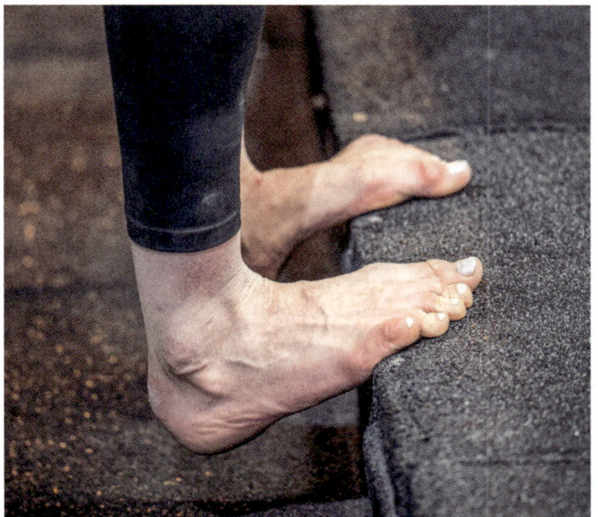

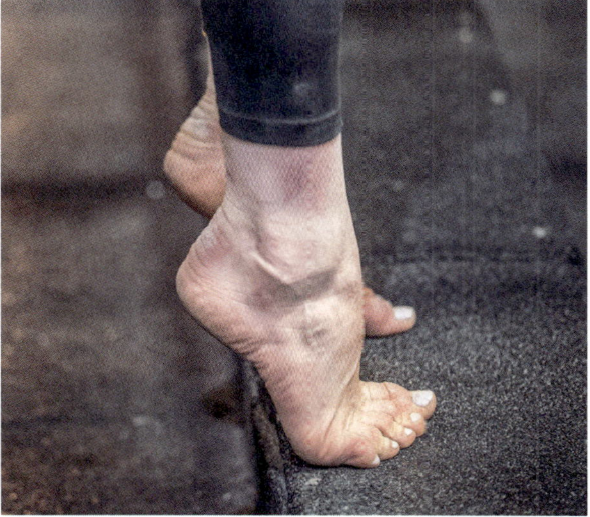

HEEL RAISE. Stand on the edge of a box, step or similar. Lower your heels past a flat position and then push all the way up on your toes. Do 8–12 repetitions, once a day.

FEET AND TOES

Two sizes down from your regular shoes. Banana-shaped and twisted towards the big toe. A heel cup that tightens over the heel and around the Achilles tendon. All to maximise pressure on the footholds, to keep the heel in place and to allow the toes to function as claws on steep terrain. Climbing shoes are not made for comfort, they are made for function. But is it really that important that they are *SO* tight? And what consequences does this have for your feet and toes?

From a personal perspective, it's important for me to have tight shoes. Mine are about 2–2½ sizes smaller than my regular shoes, and I am so used to climbing with tight shoes that it feels more uncomfortable to climb in shoes that are too big. And this is not uncommon among climbers with many years of experience and at higher levels – their climbing shoes are generally a couple of sizes smaller than their regular shoes. Not surprisingly, function is chosen over comfort, but it is important to emphasise that this absolutely does not apply to everyone. The most important thing is to have a climbing shoe that fits well on your foot and allows you to climb without pain. At lower levels, the need for stiffness, precision or feeling isn't as high as in more difficult climbing, and just like I probably don't need an alpine world cup skier's set-up to go skiing, not all climbers need high-end climbing shoes two sizes smaller than their sneakers.

Tight climbing shoes lead most climbers to report discomfort and pain in their feet and toes during climbing. There is a relationship between prolonged use of tight climbing shoes and symptoms such as skin or nail changes, joint pain and bunions, such as *hallux valgus* – a condition where the big toe angles inwards toward the middle of the foot. Since both the extent and severity of such problems seem closely related to climbing level and a reduction in shoe size, it seems obvious that reducing the time spent in very tight shoes would be a good strategy for avoiding such problems. This can be done by using more spacious and comfortable shoes for training, and by taking your shoes off regularly during a climbing session. Your tight and perfectly fitted redpoint shoes shouldn't be worn for long anyway – just long enough for you to send! A conscious approach to choosing shoes for different purposes and the amount of time you wear them for will likely contribute positively to reducing foot and toe problems throughout your climbing life.

However, some conditions may require a more comprehensive approach than just adjusting shoe size, shoe type and duration of use. In my practice, I regularly see inflammation in the base joint of the big toe and the development of bunions. While the former can be treated with cortisone injections into the joint if the inflammation doesn't improve with changes in footwear and load management, managing bunions requires an individualised approach. This ranges from relieving pressure on the big toe through taping, exercises and adaptation of footwear, all the way to surgical treatment. If you have a symptomatic bunion, I recommend contacting a healthcare professional who can help you manage this condition in the best possible way.

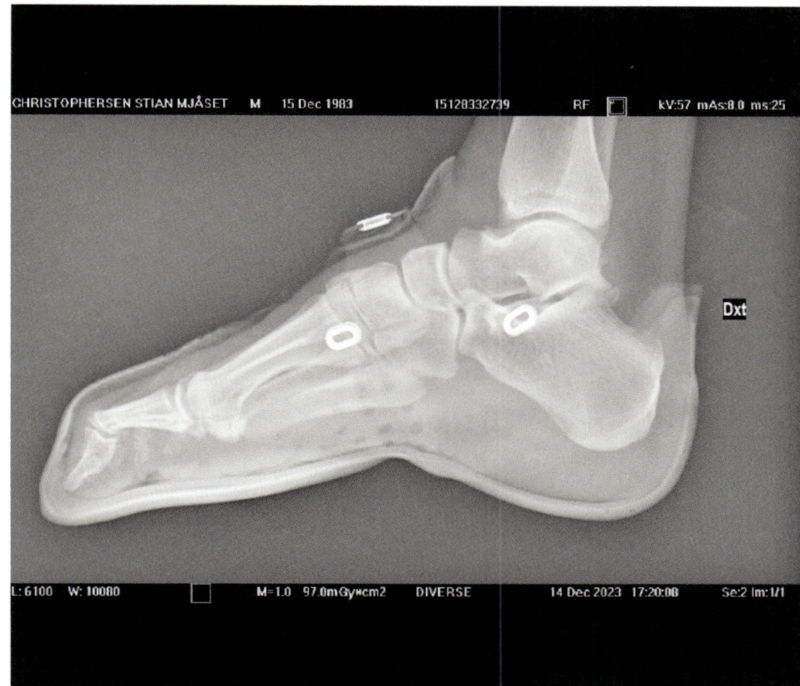

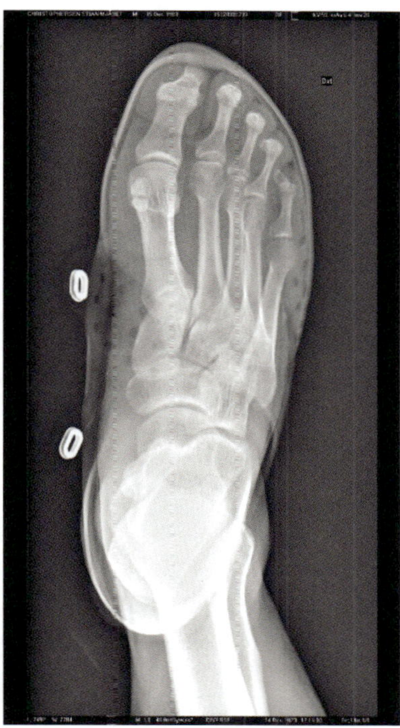

X-rays of the author's foot in a climbing shoe. Note the joint angles in the big toe and how all the toes are pressed together to transfer as much force as possible to the tip of the big toe. Thanks to Helene Lund and Unilabs Bryn for the X-rays.

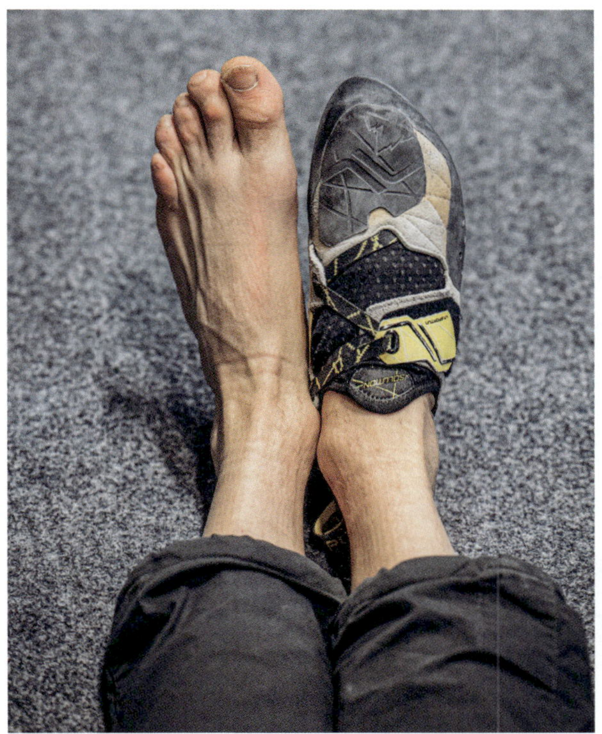

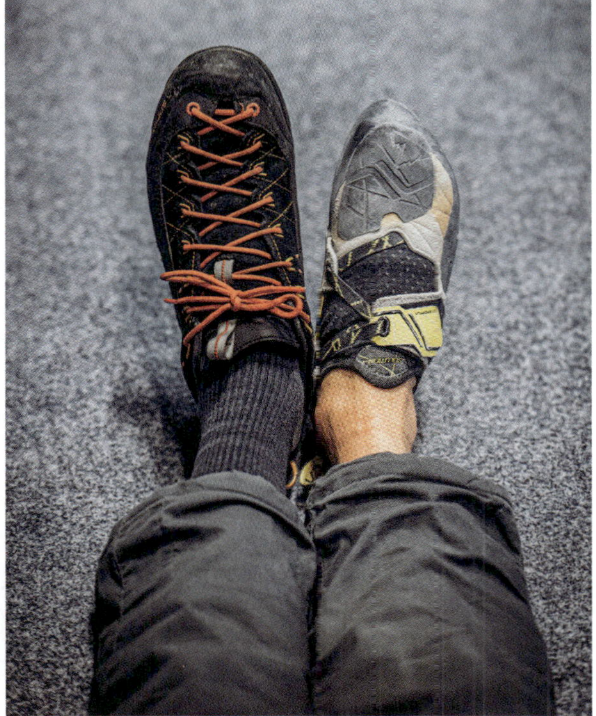

A foot with street shoe size 42 that will fit in a size 39 climbing shoe. It's natural that it's not a comfortable experience and it's not necessary for everyone, all the time. In cases where you really need a tight and precise shoe, make sure you don't wear it for longer than necessary – if you had even considered that option.

PHOTO: TERJE AAMODT

03

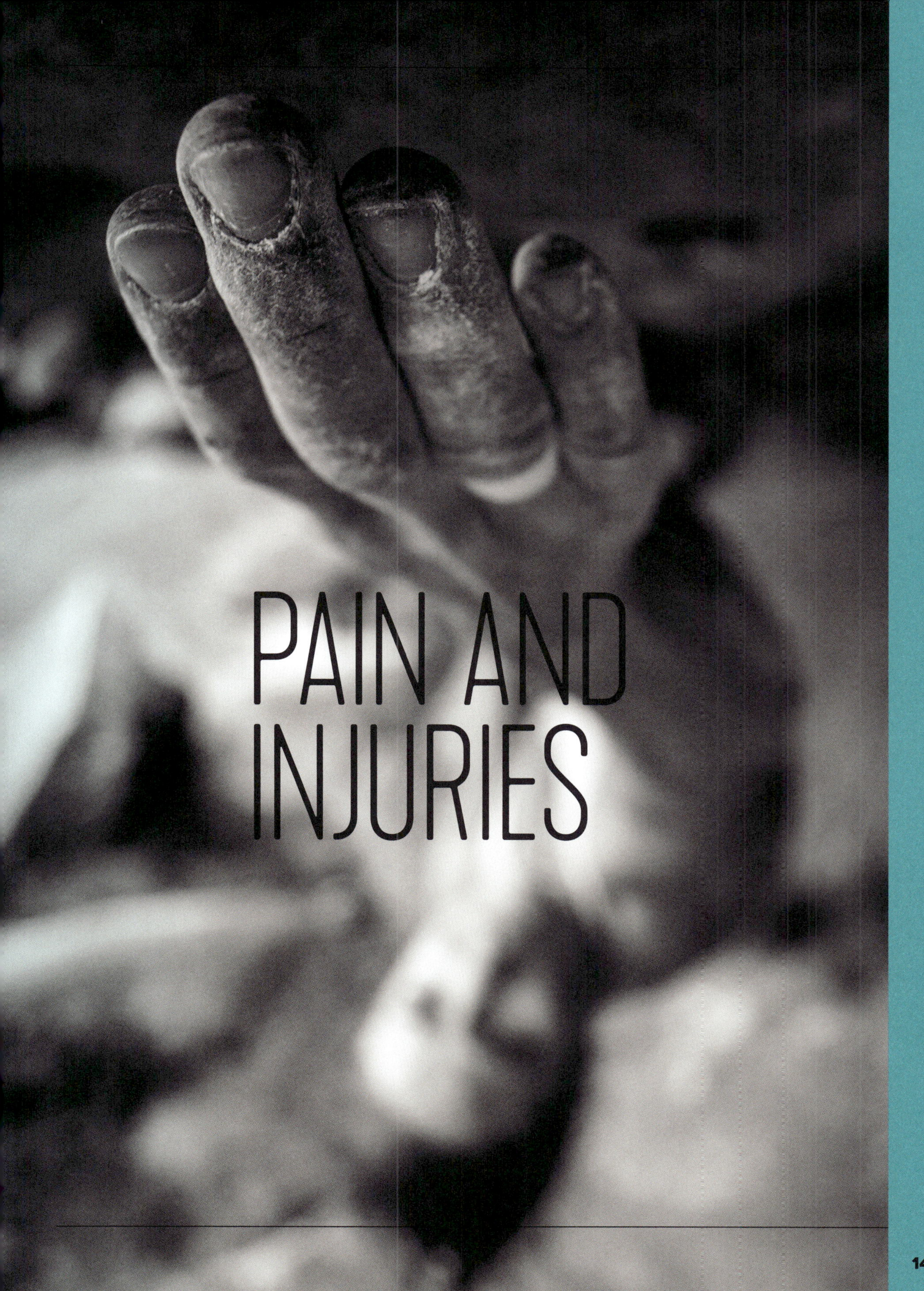

PAIN AND INJURIES

WHAT IS PAIN, REALLY?

'THE AMOUNT OF PAIN YOU EXPERIENCE DOES NOT NECESSARILY RELATE TO THE AMOUNT OF TISSUE DAMAGE YOU HAVE SUSTAINED.'

LORIMER MOSELEY

As I wrote in the introduction, when I was 16 years old, I experienced pain in both middle fingers for a long time. I woke up in pain, climbed with pain and felt it pretty much all the time over a period of about six months. No one could tell me what was causing it, and I didn't accept doctors' advice to take it easy or take a break from climbing altogether. After six months, two doctors and many terrible sessions, doctor number three explained to me that I had growth plate fractures in both fingers – *'like Schlatter's in the fingers'*, I remember him saying – and that I was going to be completely fine as long as I didn't climb for six weeks. (Osgood-Schlatter's disease is a common cause of knee pain in growing children.) Even though it was a brutal message for an ambitious young athlete to receive, I still remember that the pain in my fingers almost disappeared that day: finally, I had an answer.

But it's not like being given that answer healed the damage – the growth plates were just as broken – but my understanding of the symptoms had changed. And with a changed understanding, my pain also changed. To quote Moseley again:

'ANYTHING THAT CHANGES YOUR BRAIN'S EVALUATION OF DANGER WILL CHANGE PAIN.'

We can consider the experience of pain in the same way as the experience of seeing: colours are picked up by sensors in the retina and sent as electrical signals to the brain, which, with the help of all available information, must make sense of these signals. I think we can all agree that our visual experiences are vulnerable to errors – that is, we don't always see what we thought we saw, we see things that aren't there, or we don't see things that are actually there. The quicker we must make sense of the information, and the more stressed we are, the more vulnerable we are to misinterpretation. Similarly, nerve fibres dedicated to registering elements such as load, speed, temperature, pressure, stretch and vibration pick up signals in our tissues and send them to the brain. The brain then makes an assessment, based on numerous factors, about the extent to which we need protection. The more factors that point in the direction of danger, the greater the need for protection – and pain has always been a good indicator of danger, thus ensuring our protection.

The pain response depends on how we interpret the information we have available, and that interpretation is based on three questions:

1. Am I safe?
2. Do I have information to predict the future?
3. Do I have information to influence the future?

The safer we consider the situation to be, the less the need for protection, and thus less pain. Pain is a protective mechanism and an experience, coloured by situations we find ourselves in, and can be experienced differently in different settings based on how we interpret a situation. Most of all, it is based on how dangerous a situation is for us. And all climbers who are faced with the risk of having to climb less, climb easier or – God forbid – stop for a period, will experience this as a situation that requires both protection and action.

It is important to understand that tissue damage is not necessary for the experience of pain. It's sufficient that there is a *possible* injury, and a situation that is experienced as dangerous or threatening for the person concerned. Pain is one of the most important survival mechanisms we have, but it is overprotective by nature and vulnerable to misinterpretation. Muscle soreness is a good example – it's not just a type of pain we live well with, it's actually a pain we take pride in and which gives us satisfaction. What distinguishes this soreness from other load-related ailments? When should we challenge and push on, and when should we end the session and possibly rest? These are experiences we build throughout our lives, and thus we also must accept being in pain for periods.

When we are faced with a situation that feels dangerous, in the form of having possible consequences such as a break from climbing and, perhaps, a reduced quality of life, pain is an appropriate response until we know more about the situation. The pain response is made up by both bodily signals and how we interpret these signals, based on our own knowledge, our experiences and memories, in what context it has happened, and what consequences it may have for us. It is important to understand this so that we can see the difference between pain and injury.

SENSITISATION

A smoke alarm in your house has a crucial job. It notifies you if there is smoke from a fire in your house so that you can save both your house and your life. It is equipped with sensors that detect smoke, and if the amount of smoke becomes large enough, the alarm will go off. Sometimes, though, the alarm can go off when you are cooking or when steam comes out of the bathroom after a long, hot shower. But, in the name of safety, one time too many is better, right? Better to be safe than sorry?

Or ... ?

Unlike a smoke alarm, the human nervous system is adaptable, and can turn its sensitivity up and down. Sometimes it happens as a natural consequence of the body's condition – just think how it can hurt to touch your skin when you have a fever. Sometimes it happens as a natural consequence of the situation you find yourself in – just think how vigilant you might feel if you were to walk alone at night through a park where you knew others had been robbed. This up-regulation of sensitivity has obvious advantages for our survival, and therefore the same up-regulation will occur in response to injuries so that we don't worsen the condition. The more sensitive our warning system, the less of a stimulus required to trigger a response – in this case, pain. But what if it is not dangerous to load that body part after all? That it is rather the opposite, that we *must* load the tissues to rehabilitate an injury as best as possible? Put another way: if you like to light candles at home, it is not desirable to have a smoke alarm that goes off every time you light a match. Even though the smoke alarm has an absolutely crucial job, we must do something about the sensitivity of the system.

Sensitisation of the nervous system occurs after all types of injuries and ailments, and just being aware that pain does not always mean injury, and that our warning system naturally becomes more sensitive after an injury, can make us feel a little more confident that we can still exercise, train and climb. To get there, we need to expose ourselves to and form new positive experiences.

MOVEMENT OPTIMISM

From an evolutionary perspective, we have benefited from placing more emphasis on the negative than the positive. Avoiding something which has a potentially negative outcome gives us a greater chance of survival than seeking out the positive. Negative information is therefore weighted more heavily than positive, and this affects (among other things) attention, motivation, behaviour, physiology and decision making. This is called *negativity bias* and is certainly relevant when it comes to pain and injuries.

As previously described, the experience of pain is a protective mechanism, and when we assess the information available to us, we will to a greater extent emphasise the negative over the positive. This tendency can cause us to avoid painful movements and take a darker view of the future, which in turn leads to an even greater focus on the negative than on the positive. It is not without reason that a low degree of pain self-efficacy, catastrophising and depression are closely linked to long-term pain conditions, and it is absolutely essential that we reverse this trend in order to contribute to as short a period as possible, with the best possible outcome.

Optimism is defined as *'hopefulness and confidence about the future'*, and an optimist expects positive things to occur in their future. This may sound naive, but optimism is closely linked to health-promoting effects – both physical and psychological. Optimism is also believed to influence our experience of pain and how we cope with painful conditions, and the outcome of a number of musculoskeletal disorders is closely linked to both positive expectations and a high degree of pain self-efficacy. Looking more brightly at the future creates more hope for recovery and more positive expectations for the course of the injury. This in turn increases the likelihood that we will complete the work that needs to be done, that we will better cope with fluctuating increases in symptom response, that we will manage relapses better and that we will return to our desired level sooner.

The same injury can therefore take two completely different courses in two different people who have different attitudes. A pulley injury can be seen as something catastrophic or something that is going to go well: as an injury which has ended the season and which creates uncertainty as to whether we will ever return to the same level; or as an opportunity to experience what this injury entails, an opportunity to work on other things in our climbing, and an opportunity to try other training methods which might even take us to a new level in the future. As Irish MMA fighter Conor McGregor said, *'Injury is not just a process of recovery, it's a process of discovery.'*

It is easier to be optimistic if we are given good information and advice that creates safety and predictability, and here comes a plea to healthcare professionals out there: we must familiarise ourselves with the types of injuries we encounter in practice, and with the sports and activities people take part in and want to return to. In this way, we can give good advice, emphasise the possibilities, and adapt the training to the individual's goals and wishes. We must be aware of the language we use, so that we do not create unnecessary fear and pessimism. Many of us are trained in a tradition where we must find faults and fix them, but we have been trained to a lesser extent in how to communicate such findings and the rehabilitation plans in a positive framework. If we can become as good and confident in this as in the job of diagnosing and making training plans, we can contribute to a far more optimistic recovery from injuries, and thus to a better prognosis and outcome.

No rehabilitation process has a linear progression, and it is important that healthcare professionals and unfortunate climbers are aware of this. Being prepared for the fact that the road can be bumpy and offer both stagnation and relapse creates a more realistic expectation than believing that rehab will progress in a linear fashion from day to day. The English physiotherapist Adam Meakins has created a humorous representation of this, and I have this picture hanging in my office to help me to discuss the way forwards with those I meet at the clinic.

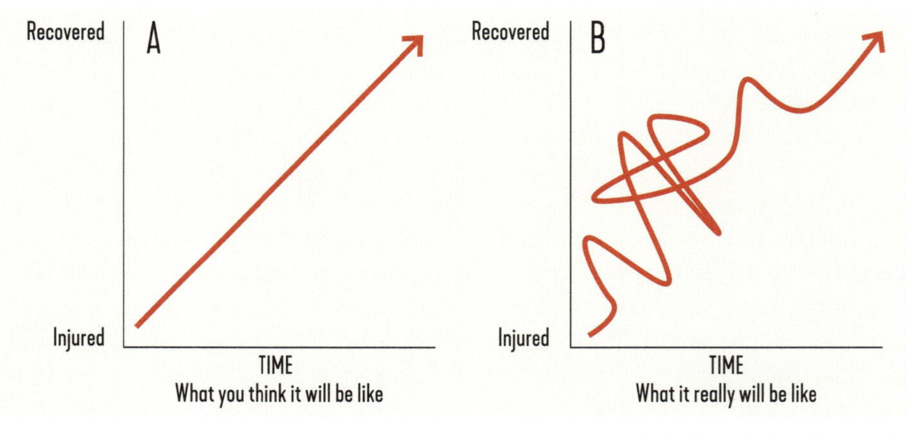

Nor is it the case that we are either an optimist or a pessimist. Being optimistic is a quality that can be trained, just like anything else. It is a conscious choice as to how we want to look at the future. Injuries are a part of sport, unfortunately, and both reducing injury risk and managing injuries are performance factors in just the same way as training to get stronger fingers. We can train to be more optimistic, and such training programmes show promising results in working with cognitive strategies for long-term pain. By thinking about and writing down the desired outcomes where everything ends well, and writing down all the possibilities we have despite the injury, the focus shifts from the negative to the positive. Some days are of course shit: we're disappointed, down and sad, and this is understandable and acceptable. But we must then try to turn the tide and work our way back to a more optimistic view of things, as this is what opens up the door to a better end result.

A term that has been introduced in recent years is *movement optimism*. Based on knowledge of an injury, we can move away from the idea that pain is the same as injury and rather see the pain as a necessary part of the learning process in a rehabilitation course. Instead of avoiding movements we are afraid of or that cause pain, we can adjust the load and make the context safer so that we can expose ourselves to these movements. In this way, we can load the tissue, but also challenge the assumption that the movement is dangerous or causes an increase in pain.

EXPOSURE

We're exposed to things all the time, and we try to predict what will happen as a consequence of the things we are exposed to. If we have been exposed to something a lot, we will have formed experiences around it and so we can use these experiences to predict what will happen if we do one thing or another. When we are exposed to something we have not experienced before, we must form new experiences, and since the negative usually outweighs the positive, it will also shape what experiences we are left with and how we think similar situations will play out in the future.

A simple example of this is touching an electric fence. The first time you touch it, you learn that it hurts to get an electric shock. This experience means that you will (perhaps) not touch an electric fence again, and thus avoid injuring yourself. Next, imagine that you are standing in front of another electric fence, but now you don't know whether it is turned on or not. How would you touch it if you had to? Of course, it depends on the situation, but in a safe environment most people would assume that they were going to get shocked, and thus be very careful about touching the fence. Your past experience means that a 50-50 situation is handled as something much, much worse, and you'd prefer to avoid a shock. Some may also have never touched an electric fence because they have heard that it hurts. They therefore don't need to have experienced something themselves to avoid a situation; it is sufficient to base their choices on the experiences of others. This also applies in the event of an injury. If we have pain somewhere and then google the symptoms, we will try to predict the future based on other people's experiences. This is rarely good when it comes to being optimistic, since we will emphasise any negative information to a greater extent than any positive information.

Most of us have been sore after training. The first few times you experienced this you were perhaps unsure what was wrong, but were reassured by the surroundings and the people around you and were told that it wasn't dangerous and would pass within a few days. It did pass, and you have most certainly repeated this cycle numerous times throughout your life. Through this exposure to the symptoms of a low-grade muscle injury, we experience that it can be unpleasant and can inhibit the quality of training that day, but that it passes without major consequences. Exposure is therefore crucial for learning, and for us to be able to make good choices in the future.

I once asked an athlete I coached if she thought it was possible to be good at sports without experiencing periods of pain. She started laughing – she thought it was impossible. When I further asked her how she dealt with it, she said something that I believe is worth repeating:

'You must be able to put the various pains in boxes that you have control over. One box for sore skin, one for signs of illness, one for muscle soreness, one for aches and pains you can train with or around, one for aches and pains you need to pay attention to and investigate further, and one for the serious aches and pains that should take you out of training.'

EXPOSURE AND SYMPTOM RESPONSE

When we return to training and climbing after an injury, it is only natural that we experience some symptoms acutely and afterwards. But how much pain is okay? This is a difficult question to answer and it differs from injury to injury. With some injuries, such as a stress fracture in the growth plate in the finger of a young climber, we allow for little to no pain, while in other cases, such as an elbow tendinopathy, we allow as much pain as is acceptable for the individual. It is not a goal in itself that exercises and loading should hurt, but once we have ruled out serious injury, we can develop an acceptance of pain during and after exercise.

The most common measure of pain is the Visual Analogue Scale (VAS), where a patient rates their pain on a scale from 0 to 10 or 0 to 100, where 0 represents no pain. Remember that this is only a subjective experience of pain intensity, and that it is not necessarily the case that higher pain intensity equals greater damage. Also, remember that the experience of pain is affected by numerous factors, and that it can therefore be difficult to know exactly what led to something being better or worse today compared to yesterday or last week.

The advantage of using VAS is that it gives us the opportunity to see the relationship between load and symptom response over time. For example, the first sets of loading a finger after a pulley injury can cause symptoms, but then get better throughout the session and remain unchanged for the next 24 hours. We can then say that we've found a balance in the relationship between loading dose and symptom response.

A sore elbow may feel good after warming up, but then become significantly worse the following day and then persist for a few more days. Then it is likely that the loading dose was greater than the available capacity.

By following this relationship between load dose and symptom response over time, we can adjust the load up and down, and at the same time see that being able to do more without symptoms getting worse is also a big step in the right direction.

Day	1	2	3	4	5	6
What	Bouldering	Routes	Bouldering	Routes	Bouldering	Bouldering
	60 min	45 min	30 min	60 min	60 min	45 min
Intensity	Low	Low	Moderate	Low	Low	Moderate
Pain 0–10	Before: 2	Before: 2	Before: 2	Before: 2	Before: 1	Before: 1
	After: 4	After: 3	After: 4	After: 2	After: 2	After: 3

By using a training log, we can see what and how hard we have trained and monitor the pain response. It is common to measure the pain response on a scale from 0–10 where 0 equals no pain and 10 is the worst pain imaginable. Increased load usually results in an increased response, but if the pain returns to baseline during the following 24 hours, it is okay and we can continue the training. Gradually, we will be able to tolerate more load and see that the pain response decreases. On the other hand, in the event of a gradually increasing pain response, because of a too high training load, we can adjust the load down so that the trend doesn't become negative.

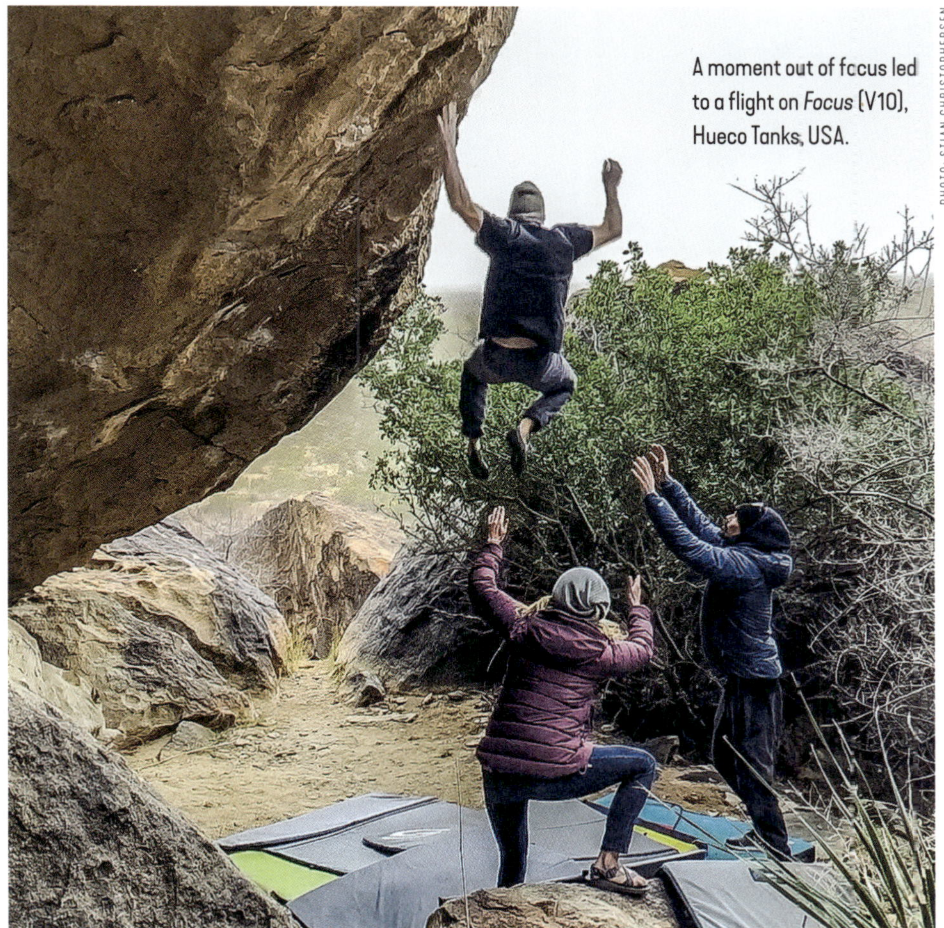

A moment out of focus led to a flight on *Focus* (V10), Hueco Tanks, USA.

PHOTO: STIAN CHRISTOPHERSEN

Feeling a little bruised after a bouldering session outdoors is not so strange, given all the times we fall off during these sessions. These are symptoms we've become accustomed to and know will pass with a little movement and time. How do these symptoms differ from other symptoms? Is it just that we've become accustomed to them, while we're unsure what the burgeoning pain in the elbow means?

When we talk about how movement optimism and exposure affect pain, it is not to trivialise an injury or to claim that one should only think positively. But in many cases, we can probably intentionally dedramatise a good number of injuries and pain conditions. In this way, we can expose ourselves to movements that can be both scary and painful, so that we can create new experiences that, through successfully completing them, hopefully create optimism and faith that things will go well. A pulley injury, a hamstring injury or a painful elbow will naturally hurt when we load it. The million dollar question then becomes what that pain *means*. If we have control over the load that we expose the tissue to, we can at least state that we are not close to the forces that can damage the tissue. If we have control over the symptom response over time, we can be sure that we are balancing the load in a good way. And if we can work with movements that we're a bit scared of and preferably want to avoid, we can create new experiences and new predictions.

Maybe there was no electricity in the fence after all?

GLOSSARY

Abduction: A movement away from the midline of the body, for example, moving your arm out to the side.

Acute: Refers to an injury with a sudden onset.

Adduction: A movement towards the midline of the body, for example, moving your arm towards the body during a pull-up.

Anterior: Front.

Campus board: A training device made up of a ladder of wooden rungs on an overhanging plywood wall.

Chronic: Refers to an injury related to overuse, which develops over time.

Concentric: The shortening of a muscle.

Crimp: Crimping involves an acute angle in the PIP joints, hyperextended DIP joints and the thumb placed over the index finger to lock the grip down.

Deadhang: A finger strength training method where you hang from the edges of a fingerboard or similar.

DIP joint: Distal interphalangeal joint. The outermost joint of the finger.

Distal: A part of the body that is farther away from the centre of the body than another part.

Dorsal: Back side. For example, the back, back of the hand, top of the foot. Dorsiflexion then implies movement towards the back side.

Eccentric: The lengthening of a muscle while it's contracting. Lengthening under tension.

Fingerboard: A board with a selection of edges and holds for training arm and finger strength.

Grip tool: A portable device to train finger strength (but can also be used to train other body areas as well).

Growth plate: The growth plate is the cartilaginous portion of long bones where the longitudinal growth of the bone takes place.

Half crimp: Grip position where the PIP joints are flexed at approximately 90 degrees.

Inflammation: A normal part of the body's response to injury or infection. Inflammation occurs when the body releases chemicals that trigger an immune response to fight off infection or heal damaged tissue.

Isometric: A static contraction.

Lateral: Outside.

Load: A broad term. In training it involves the total volume and intensity during an exercise, and involves both the external load (i.e. amount of kilograms lifted) and the internal load (i.e. how we respond to the training).

Load cell: A sensor that measures the mechanical force applied to the system.

MCP joint: Metacarpophalangeal joint. The joint at the base of the finger, where it meets the palm.

Medial: Inside.

No-hang: No-hang means, as the name suggests, that rather than hanging from the edges, you are standing on the ground and pressing your fingertips against a grip surface.

NSAIDs: Non-steroidal anti-inflammatory drugs – generally no longer recommended in the treatment of acute soft tissue injuries.

Open hand: All grip positions where the angle of the PIP joints is greater than 90 degrees.

Overcoming isometrics: Pushing, pulling or curling against a fixed object, trying to move it.

PIP joint: Proximal interphalangeal joint. The middle joint of the finger.

Posterior: Back.

Pronation: The rotation of the palm of the hand so the inner part faces down.

Proximal: A part of the body that is closer to the centre of the body than another part.

Rate of force development (RFD): A measure of how quickly a muscle can go from zero to maximum force and an important attribute of the muscles in the forearm for all kinds of climbing.

Relative Energy Deficiency in Sport (REDs): A condition of energy deficiency which causes adverse effects on all bodily systems.

Rotator cuff: A collection of four muscles – supraspinatus, subscapularis, infraspinatus and teres minor – with their associated tendons that attach as a cuff around the head of the upper arm at the shoulder.

Supination: The rotation of the palm so the inner part faces up.

Synovitis: Inflammation of the synovial membrane due to high stress within a joint.

Tendinopathy: Pain and dysfunction in a tendon, defined as a failed healing response of the tendon.

Tendonitis: Inflammation of a tendon.

Tenosynovitis: An inflammatory condition affecting the tendon sheath.

Volar: The palm side of the hand.

INJURY MANAGEMENT

Scialoia, D. and Swartzendruber, A.J., 'The R.I.C.E Protocol Is a MYTH: A Review and Recommendations', *The Sport Journal*, 24 (2020).

Rivas, F., 'In this Issue: Inflammation', *Cell*, 140/6 (2010).

Dubois, B. and Esculier, J-F., 'Soft-tissue injuries simply need PEACE and LOVE', *British Journal of Sports Medicine*, 54/2 (2020).

TRENDS IN CLIMBING INJURIES

Lutter, C., Tischer, T., Hotfiel, T., Frank, L., Enz, A., Simon, M., and Schöffl, V., 'Current Trends in Sport Climbing Injuries after the Inclusion into the Olympic Program. Analysis of 633 Injuries within the years 2017/18', *Muscle Ligaments and Tendons Journal*, 10/2 (2020).

Schöffl, V., Schöffl, I., Lutter, C. and Hochholzer, T., eds., *Climbing Medicine. A Practical Guide* (Springer, 2022).

Cole, K.P., Uhl, R.L. and Rosenbaum, A.J., 'Comprehensive Review of Rock Climbing Injuries', *Journal of the American Academy of Orthopaedic Surgeons*, 28/12 (2020).

INJURY PREVENTION

Charest, J. and Grandner, M.A., 'Sleep and Athletic Performance: Impacts on Physical Performance, Mental Performance, Injury Risk and Recovery, and Mental Health: An Update', *Sleep Medicine Clinics*, 17/2 (2022).

Impellizzeri, F.M., Menaspà, P., Coutts, A.J., Kalkhoven, J. and Menaspà, M.J., 'Training Load and Its Role in Injury Prevention, Part I: Back to the Future', *Journal of Athletic Training*, 55/9 (2020).

Dalen-Lorentsen, T., Bjørneboe, J., Clarsen, B., Vagle, M., Fagerland, M.W. and Andersen, T.E., 'Does Load Management using the Acute:Chronic Workload Ratio Prevent Health Problems? A Cluster Randomised Trial of 482 Elite Youth Footballers of Both Sexes', *British Journal of Sports Medicine*, 55/2 (2021).

Cook, J.L. and Docking, S.I., '"Rehabilitation will Increase the 'Capacity' of Your ... Insert Musculoskeletal Tissue Here ... " Defining 'Tissue Capacity': A Core Concept for Clinicians', *British Journal of Sports Medicine*, 49/23 (2015).

Glasgow, P., Phillips, N. and Bleakley, C., 'Optimal Loading: Key Variables and Mechanisms', *British Journal of Sports Medicine*, 49/5 (2015).

Emery, C.A. and Pasanen, K., 'Current Trends in Sport Injury Prevention', *Best Practice & Research Clinical Rheumatology*, 33/1 (2019).

Hottenrott, L., Ketelhut, S., Schneider, C., Wiewelhove, T. and Ferrauti, A., 'Age- and Sex-Related Differences in Recovery From High-Intensity and Endurance Exercise: A Brief Review', *International Journal of Sports Physiology and Performance*, 16/6 (2021).

Martínez-Fortuny, N., Alonso-Calvete, A., Da Cuña-Carrera, I. and Abalo-Núñez, R., 'Menstrual Cycle and Sport Injuries: A Systematic Review', *International Journal of Environmental Research and Public Health*, 20/4 (2023).

PULLEYS

Schöffl, V., Schöffl, I., Lutter, C. and Hochholzer, T., eds., *Climbing Medicine. A Practical Guide* (Springer, 2022).

Schweizer, A., 'Biomechanics of the Interaction of Finger Flexor Tendons and Pulleys in Rock Climbing', *Sports Technology*, 1/6 (2008).

Schneeberger, M. and Schweizer, A., 'Pulley Ruptures in Rock Climbers: Outcome of Conservative Treatment With the Pulley-Protection Splint-A Series of 47 Cases', *Wilderness & Environmental Medicine*, 27/2 (2016).

Larsson, R., Nordeman, L. and Blomdahl, C., 'To Tape or Not to Tape: Annular Ligament (Pulley) Injuries in Rock Climbers – A Systematic Review', *BMC Sports Science, Medicine and Rehabilitation*, 14 (2022).

Schöffl, V., Schöffl, I., Frank, L. Küpper, T., Simon, M. and Lutter, C., 'Tendon Injuries in the Hands in Rock Climbers: Epidemiology, Anatomy, Biomechanics and Treatment – An Update', *Muscle Ligaments and Tendons Journal*, 10/2 (2020).

TENOSYNOVITIS

Mohn, S., Spörri, J., Mauler, F., Kabelitz, M. and Schweizer, A., 'Nonoperative Treatment of Finger Flexor Tenosynovitis in Sport Climbers – A Retrospective Descriptive Study Based on a Clinical 10-Year Database', *Biology*, 11/6 (2022).

Muthu, S., Annamalai, S. and Kandasamy, V., 'Tenosynovitis of Hand: Causes and Complications', *World Journal of Clinical Cases*, 12/4 (2024).

Schöffl, V., Strohm, P. and Lutter, C., 'Efficacy of Corticosteroid Injection in Rock Climber's Tenosynovitis', *Hand Surgery and Rehabilitation*, 38/5 (2019).

FINGER JOINTS

Vagy, J., 'Clinical Management of Finger Joint Capsulitis/Synovitis in a Rock Climber', *Frontiers in Sports and Active Living*, 5 (2023).

Pastor, T., Schweizer, A., Andronic, O., Dietrich, L.G., Berk, T., Gueorguiev, B. and Pastor, T., 'A Life Dedicated to Climbing and Its Sequelae in the Fingers – A Review of the Literature', *International Journal of Environmental Research and Public Health*, 19/24 (2022).

Pastor, T., Fröhlich, S., Spörri, J., Schreiber, T. and Schweizer, A., 'Cartilage Abnormalities and Osteophytes in the Fingers of Elite Sport Climbers: An Ultrasonography-based Cross-Sectional Study', *European Journal of Sport Science*, 20/2 (2020).

GROWTH PLATES

Garcia, K., Jaramillo, D. and Rubesova, E., 'Ultrasound Evaluation of Stress Injuries and Physiological Adaptations in the Fingers of Adolescent Competitive Rock Climbers', *Pediatric Radiology*, 48/3 (2018).

Lutter, C., Tischer, T. and Schöffl V.R., 'Olympic Competition Climbing: the Beginning of a New Era – A Narrative Review', *British Journal of Sports Medicine*, 55/15 (2021).

Schöffl, V., Schöffl, I., Flohé, S., El-Sheikh, Y. and Lutter, C., 'Evaluation of a Diagnostic-Therapeutic Algorithm for Finger Epiphyseal Growth Plate Stress Injuries in Adolescent Climbers', *The American Journal of Sports Medicine*, 50/1 (2022).

Bärtschi, N., Scheibler, A. and Schweizer, A., 'Symptomatic Epiphyseal Sprains and Stress Fractures of the Finger Phalanges in Adolescent Sport Climbers', *Hand Surgery and Rehabilitation*, 38/4 (2019).

Schöffl, I. and Schöffl, V., 'Epiphyseal Stress Fractures in the Fingers of Adolescents: Biomechanics, Pathomechanism, and Risk Factors', *European Journal of Sports Medicine*, 3/1 (2015).

Schweizer, A. and Göhner Schweizer, K. 'Sportklettern, Bouldern und Assoziierte Verletzungen im Kindes- und Jugendalter [Sport Climbing, Bouldering and Associated Injuries in Childhood and Adolescence]', *Der Orthopade*, 48/12 (2019).

Borchsenius, C., 'Har du hørt om REDs? [Have you heard of REDs?]', Sunn Idrett [Healthy Sports], https://sunnidrett.no/har-du-hort-om-red-s

Dudgeon, E., 'Relative energy deficiency in sport (RED-S): recognition and next steps', BMJ blog (22 April 2019), https://blogs.bmj.com/bjsm/2019/04/22/relative-energy-deficiency-in-sport-red-s-recognition-and-next-steps

FLEXOR MUSCLES, LUMBRICALS AND DUPUYTREN'S CONTRACTURE

Schöffl, V., Heid, A. and Küpper, T., 'Tendon Injuries of the Hand', *World Journal of Orthopedics*, 3/6 (2012).

Wang, E.H., Loftus, W.K., Bird, S.J. and Sampson, M.J., 'Ring Finger Lumbrical Origin Strain: A Case Series with Imaging Findings', *Skeletal Radiology*, 45/12 (2016).

Dutta, A., Jayasinghe, G., Deore, S., Wahed, K., Bhan, K., Bakti, N. and Singh, B., 'Dupuytren's Contracture – Current Concepts', *Journal of Clinical Orthopaedics and Trauma*, 11/4 (2020).

Hamilton, B., Alonso, J.M. and Best, T.M., 'Best Time for a Paradigm Shift in the Classification of Muscle Injuries', *Journal of Sport and Health Science*, 6/3 (2017).

Pollock, N., James, S.L.J., Lee, J.C. and Chakraverty, R., 'British Athletics Muscle Injury Classification: A New Grading System', *British Journal of Sports Medicine*, 48/18 (2014).

SHOULDERS

Hegedus, E.J., Cook, C., Lewis, J., Wright, A. and Park, J.Y., 'Combining Orthopedic Special Tests to Improve Diagnosis of Shoulder Pathology', *Physical Therapy in Sport*, 16/2 (2015).

Brownson, P., Donaldson, O., Fox, M., Rees, J.L., Rangan, A., Jaggi, A., Tytherleigh-Strong, G., McBernie, J., Thomas, M. and Kulkarni, R., 'BESS/BOA Patient Care Pathways: Traumatic Anterior Shoulder Instability', *Shoulder & Elbow*, 7/3 (2015).

Noorani, A., Goldring, M., Jaggi, A., Gibson, J., Rees, J., Bateman, M., Falworth, M. and Brownson, P., 'BESS/BOA Patient Care Pathways: Atraumatic Shoulder Instability', *Shoulder & Elbow*, 11/1 (2019).

Gooding, B.W.T., Geoghegan, J.M. and Manning, P.A., 'The Management of Acute Traumatic Primary Anterior Shoulder Dislocation in Young Adults', *Shoulder & Elbow*, 2/3 (2010).

Kavaja, L., Lähdeoja, T., Malmivaara, A. and Paavola, M., 'Treatment after Traumatic Shoulder Dislocation: A Systematic Review with a Network Meta-analysis', *British Journal of Sports Medicine*, 52/23 (2018).

King, S.W. and Cowling, P.D., 'Management of First Time Shoulder Dislocation', *Journal of Arthroscopy and Joint Surgery*, 5/2 (2018).

Hurley, E.T., Manjunath, A.K., Bloom, D.A., Pauzenberger, L., Mullett, H., Alaia, M.J. and Strauss, E.J., 'Arthroscopic Bankart Repair Versus Conservative Management for First-Time Traumatic Anterior Shoulder Instability: A Systematic Review and Meta-analysis', *Arthroscopy*, 36/9 (2020).

Girish, G., Lobo, L.G., Jacobson, J.A., Morag, Y., Miller, B. and Jamadar, D.A., 'Ultrasound of the Shoulder: Asymptomatic Findings in Men', *American Journal of Roentgenology*, 197/4 (2011).

Barreto, R.P.G., Braman, J.P., Ludewig, P.M., Ribeiro, L.P. and Camargo, P.R., 'Bilateral Magnetic Resonance Imaging Findings in Individuals with Unilateral Shoulder Pain', *Journal of Shoulder and Elbow Surgery*, 28/9 (2019).

Rahu, M., Kolts, I., Põldoja, E. and Kask, K., 'Rotator Cuff Tendon Connections with the Rotator Cable', *Knee Surgery, Sports Traumatology, Arthroscopy*, 25/7 (2016).

LeVasseur, M.R., Mancini, M.R., Hawthorne, B.C., Romeo, A.A., Calvo, E. and Mazzocca, A.D., 'SLAP Tears and Return to Sport and Work: Current Concepts', *Journal of ISAKOS*, 6/4 (2021).

Liaghat, B., Pedersen, J.R., Husted, R.S., Pedersen, L.L., Thorborg, K. and Juhl, C.B., 'Diagnosis, Prevention and Treatment of Common Shoulder Injuries in Sport: Grading the Evidence – A Statement Paper Commissioned by the Danish Society of Sports Physical Therapy (DSSF)', *British Journal of Sports Medicine*, 57/7 (2023).

Schrøder, C.P., Skare, Ø., Reikerås, O., Mowinckel, P. and Brox, J.I., 'Sham Surgery Versus Labral Repair or Biceps Tenodesis for Type II SLAP Lesions of the Shoulder: A Three-armed Randomised Clinical Trial', *British Journal of Sports Medicine*, 51/24 (2017).

Cuff, A. and Littlewood, C., 'Subacromial Impingement Syndrome – What Does this Mean to and for the Patient? A Qualitative Study', *Musculoskeletal Science & Practice*, 33 (2018).

Chester, R., Jerosch-Herold, C., Lewis, J. and Shepstone, L., 'Psychological Factors are Associated with the Outcome of Physiotherapy for People with Shoulder Pain: A Multicentre Longitudinal Cohort Study', *British Journal of Sports Medicine*, 52/4 (2018).

Chester, R., Khondoker, M., Shepstone, L., Lewis, J.S. and Jerosch-Herold, C., 'Self-efficacy and Risk of Persistent Shoulder Pain: Results of a Classification and Regression Tree (CART) Analysis', *British Journal of Sports Medicine*, 53/13 (2019).

ELBOWS

van Middelkoop, M., Bruens, M.L., Coert, J.H., Selles, R.W., Verhagen, E., Bierma-Zeinstra, S.M.A. and Koes, B.W., 'Incidence and Risk Factors for Upper Extremity Climbing Injuries in Indoor Climbers', *International Journal of Sports Medicine*, 36/10 (2015).

Sims, L.A., 'Upper Extremity Injuries in Rock Climbers: Diagnosis and Management', *The Journal of Hand Surgery*, 47/7 (2022).

Bollen, S.R., 'Soft Tissue Injury in Extreme Rock Climbers', *British Journal of Sports Medicine*, 22/4 (1988).

TENDINOPATHY

Bohm, S., Mersmann, F. and Arampatzis, A., 'Functional Adaptation of Connective Tissue by Training', *Deutsche Zeitschrift für Sportmedizin*, 70 (2019).

Cardoso, T.B., Pizzari, T., Kinsella, R., Hope, D. and Cook, J.L., 'Current Trends in Tendinopathy Management', *Best Practice & Research Clinical Rheumatology*, 33/1 (2019).

Ackermann, P.W., Alim, M.A., Pejler, G. and Peterson, M., 'Tendon Pain – What are the Mechanisms Behind It?' *Scandinavian Journal of Pain*, 23/1 (2022).

Cook, J.L. and Docking, S.I., '"Rehabilitation will Increase the 'Capacity' of Your ... Insert Musculoskeletal Tissue Here ... " Defining 'Tissue Capacity': A Core Concept for Clinicians', *British Journal of Sports Medicine*, 49/23 (2015).

Baar, K., 'Minimizing Injury and Maximizing Return to Play: Lessons from Engineered Ligaments', *Sports Medicine*, 47/1 (2017).

Baar, K., 'Stress Relaxation and Targeted Nutrition to Treat Patellar Tendinopathy', *International Journal of Sport Nutrition and Exercise Metabolism*, 29/4 (2019).

WRIST

Jawed, A., Ansari, M.T. and Gupta, V., 'TFCC Injuries: How We Treat?' *Journal of Clinical Orthopaedics and Trauma*, 11/4 (2020).

Lutter, C., Schweizer, A., Hochholzer, T., Bayer, T. and Schöffl, V., 'Pulling Harder than the Hamate Tolerates: Evaluation of Hamate Injuries in Rock Climbing and Bouldering', *Wilderness & Environmental Medicine*, 27/4 (2016).

Sander, A.L., Sommer, K., Kaiser, A.K., Marzi, I. and Frank, J., 'Outcome of Conservative Treatment for Triangular Fibrocartilage Complex Lesions with Stable Distal Radioulnar Joint', *European Journal of Trauma and Emergency Surgery*, 47/5 (2021).

Schöffl, V., von Schroeder, H., Lisse, J., El-Sheikh, Y., Küpper, T., Klinder, A. and Lutter, C., 'Wrist Injuries in Climbers', *The American Journal of Sports Medicine*, 51/13 (2023).

Dorich, J.M. and Cornwall, R., 'Evaluation of a Grip-Strengthening Algorithm for the Initial Treatment of Chronic, Nonspecific Wrist Pain in Adolescents', *Journal of Hand Surgery Global Online*, 4/1 (2021).

KNEE

Lutter, C., Tischer, T., Cooper, C., Frank, L., Hotfiel, T., Lenz, R. and Schöffl, V., 'Mechanisms of Acute Knee Injuries in Bouldering and Rock Climbing Athletes', *The American Journal of Sports Medicine*, 48/3 (2020).

HAMSTRING

Vantorre, A. and Schellhammer, F., 'Severe Injuries of Proximal Hamstrings in High-Performance Sport Climbers', *Deutsche Zeitschrift für Sportmedizin*, 73 (2022).

Ehiogu, U.D., Stephens, G., Jones, G. and Schöffl, V., 'Acute Hamstring Muscle Tears in Climbers – Current Rehabilitation Concepts', *Wilderness & Environmental Medicine*, 31/4 (2020).

Schöffl, V., Lutter, C. and Popp, D., 'The "Heel Hook" – A Climbing-Specific Technique to Injure the Leg', *Wilderness & Environmental Medicine*, 27/2 (2016).

ANKLE AND FOOT

Schöffl, V. and Küpper, T., 'Feet Injuries in Rock Climbers', *World Journal of Orthopedics*, 4/4 (2013).

Lejonagoitia-Garmendia, M., Gustran-Iglesias, I., Gil, S.M., Ortuondo, J., Sarasola-Ruiz, L. and Bidaurrazaga-Letona, I., 'Foot Injuries in Sport Climbers: Footwear and other Associated Factors', *Revista Internacional de Medicina y Ciencias de la Actividad Física y el Deporte*, 23/90 (2023).

Cobos-Moreno, P., Astasio-Picado, Á. and Gómez-Martín, B., 'Epidemiological Study of Foot Injuries in the Practice of Sport Climbing', *International Journal of Environmental Research and Public Health*, 19/7 (2022).

PAIN, EXPOSURE AND MOVEMENT OPTIMISM

Moseley, L. and Butler, D.S., *Explain Pain Supercharged* (NOI Group Publications, 2017).

Goodin, B.R. and Bulls, H.W., 'Optimism and the Experience of Pain: Benefits of Seeing the Glass as Half Full', *Current Pain and Headache Reports*, 17/5 (2013).

Norris, C.J., 'The Negativity Bias, Revisited: Evidence from Neuroscience Measures and an Individual Differences Approach', *Social Neuroscience*, 16/1 (2021).

Leemans, L., Nijs, J., Antonis, L., Wideman, T.H., Bandt, H.D., Franklin, Z., Mullie, P., Moens, M., Joos, E. and Beckwée, D., 'Do Psychological Factors Relate to Movement-evoked Pain in People with Musculoskeletal Pain? A Systematic Review and Meta-analysis', *Brazilian Journal of Physical Therapy*, 26/6 (2022).

De Baets, L., Matheve, T., Meeus, M., Struyf, F. and Timmermans, A., 'The Influence of Cognitions, Emotions and Behavioral Factors on Treatment Outcomes in Musculoskeletal Shoulder Pain: A Systematic Review', *Clinical Rehabilitation*, 33/6 (2019).

Flink, I., Reme, S., Jacobsen, H., Glombiewski, J., Vlaeyen, J., Nicholas, M., Main, C., Peters, M., Williams, A., Schrooten, M., Shaw, W. and Boersma, K., 'Pain Psychology in the 21st Century: Lessons Learned and Moving Forward', *Scandinavian Journal of Pain*, 20/2 (2020).

Meulders, A., 'From Fear of Movement-related Pain and Avoidance to Chronic Pain Disability: A State-of-the-Art Review', *Current Opinion in Behavioral Sciences*, 26 (2019)

Seymour, B., 'Pain: A Precision Signal for Reinforcement Learning and Control', *Neuron*, 101/6 (2019).

BOOKS

Mobråten, M. and Christophersen, S., *The Climbing Bible* (Vertebrate Publishing, 2020).

Mobråten, M. and Christophersen, S., *The Climbing Bible: Practical Exercises* (Vertebrate Publishing, 2022)

Feehally, N., *Beastmaking* (Vertebrate Publishing, 2021).

Moffatt, J., *Mastermind* (Vertebrate Publishing, 2022).

Consuegra, S., *The Science of Climbing Training* (Vertebrate Publishing, 2023).

McVittie, A., *The Self-Rehabbed Climber* (2022).

Vagy, J., *Climb Injury-Free* (2017).

ACKNOWLEDGEMENTS

This is a book I never thought I would write. When Vertebrate Publishing approached me two years ago, my immediate response was no. After working in the field for over 15 years, I still find it difficult to write about something so large and complex in a simple and understandable way, without making it too simple. On top of that, there are so many different opinions about the diagnosis and treatment of injuries, and not least about how we can best help people with injuries and pain. It just seemed easier not to do it. But then I read *2070*, by Norwegian climate scientist Bjørn Samset, and realised that if someone could write so well about something that is even more complex, with even more differing opinions, it was worth trying. I realised that gathering the knowledge that is out there, combined with my own and others' experiences, could be an important contribution to the growing climbing community. I also realised that the book could help climbers around the world understand and manage their own injuries and conditions, as well as stimulate further discussion and thought that could ultimately move the field forwards. It's ambitious and feels a bit like putting your head on the chopping block, but as Ted Lasso put it so well: *'If you're comfortable with what you're doing, you're doing it wrong.'*

For those of us who work with patients, it is fundamental to be able to see people with injuries and illnesses from a *biopsychosocial perspective*. An injury has its obvious biological elements, such as inflammation and tissue structure, but it also affects and is affected by psychosocial elements such as thoughts, emotions and social belonging. What makes working with people so exciting and rewarding is being able to explore all of these elements so that the way forwards can be best *individualised*. To the best of my ability, I have tried to explain how basic factors such as sleep, stress, diet, total workload, age and gender affect both the risk of injury and the management of injury. I have tried to describe the injuries I see most often in the clinic in a way that gives you a better understanding of what happened to you or the climber sitting in front of you in your clinic. I have tried to show that pain is a much more complex experience than we often realise. And, most importantly, I had a deep desire to write a book about injury in the most positive way possible. I have read enough books and research articles, and met enough people with injuries and conditions, to be convinced that optimism is a fundamental flaw in both the way knowledge is communicated and the way the situation of the injured climber is experienced. I sincerely hope that after reading this book you will have learned enough to make it a little less likely that you will be injured, and that you will have a slightly brighter outlook on life when faced with an injury.

There are many people I would like to thank for everything they have contributed to this process:

Tina Johnsen Hafsaas, Regine Storå and Joakim Louis Sæther for being my models.

Bård Lie Henriksen, for being the best photographer I could wish for.

Jon Tore Modell and Elisabet Skårberg at Redaksjonslaboratoriet AS, for turning words into pictures and creating the visual impression I wanted.

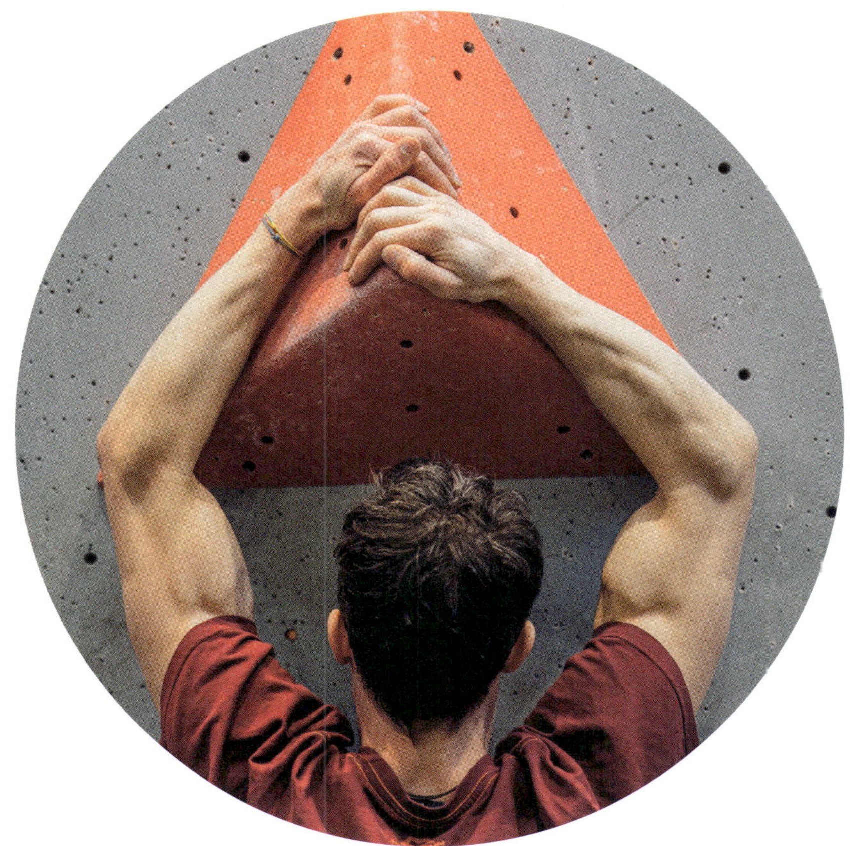

James Walker, Yngve Røe and Martin Mobråten for all their professional input, discussions and reflections.

Maria Stangeland and Marie Stenbeck-Askheim, for valuable feedback on language, content and explanatory models.

Joanna Butler, for medical illustrations.

John Coefield and Vertebrate Publishing for challenging me and believing in the project from the beginning.

I would also like to thank Mathieu Ceron, Steward Watson, Volker Schöffl, Tyler Nelson, Paul Houghoughi and Andy McVittie. You are all sources of inspiration to me and important contributors to the field as a whole. Thank you for sharing your knowledge and for being great discussion partners!

Last but not least, thank you to the climbing community, which has given me so much. This is my attempt to give something back.

Happy climbing!

THE 10 COMMANDMENTS OF CLIMBING

1. You have to climb a lot to become a good climber.
2. Vary your climbing between different styles and angles – both indoors and outdoors.
3. Train technique before physical training.
4. Learn to use your feet – they will be your best friends on the wall.
5. Rid yourself of your fear of falling.
6. Train finger strength.
7. Find your strengths and weaknesses, set yourself targets and adapt your training accordingly.
8. What and how you think is critical to your success – become just as strong mentally as you are physically and technically.
9. Create – or become part of – a supportive and challenging community.
10. Preserve the joy – climbing is all fun and games.

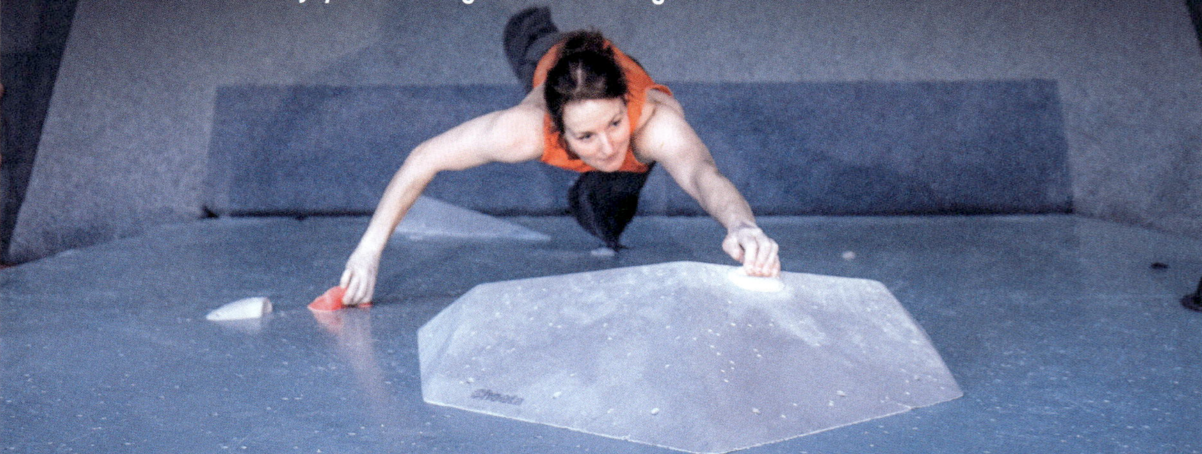